THE IMPACT OF

VITAMIN D DEFICIENCY

By Eugene L Heyden, RN

Impact Health Publishing

Spokane WA, USA

© 2014

Impact Health Publishing
Spokane, WA USA

ISBN: 978-0-9828276-1-1

Printed in the United States of America

~ For Toni ~

~*Contents*~

~*Preface*~

This book was written to share with you the importance of vitamin D and the consequences of its deficiency. You may already be aware of the fact that sunlight has been our primary source of vitamin D throughout the ages. Yet, even though the sun is all around us, in our modern society we are currently experiencing an epidemic of vitamin D deficiency. I almost hate to use the word vitamin here, as our discussion will be of a hormone, a hormone that regulates the expression of a multitude of genes. Of course, regulating genes automatically means regulating genetic events, and the genetic events targeted by vitamin D are those that maintain health, prevent disease, and promote healing. It is doubtful that you would enjoy diseases such as multiple sclerosis, cancer, diabetes, Crohn's disease, or cardiovascular disease—and did I mention cancer? No. These diseases are not attractive in the least, but they are so prevalent and so willing to destroy. However, they can, to a surprising degree, be prevented by a life that is sufficient in vitamin D. It is time you learned what this vitamin, this hormone, is all about. Now is a *great* time.

~*Eugene L. Heyden, RN*

Introduction

Vitamin D deficiency and its consequences are extremely subtle, but have enormous implications for human health and disease. **~Holick, 2003**

Vitamin D inadequacy constitutes a largely unrecognized epidemic in many populations worldwide.

Despite evidence of its profound importance to human health, vitamin D inadequacy is not widely recognized as a problem by physicians and patients. **~Holick, 2006**

Why should we care about vitamin D deficiency? <u>*It is*</u> <u>*insidious*</u> *and has both short- and long-term consequences. Infants and young children who are vitamin D deficient may be imprinted for the rest of their lives with increased risks for type I diabetes, multiple sclerosis, rheumatoid arthritis, and many common cancers. Adults are at increased risk of common cancers and cardiovascular disease.* **~Holick, 2004a, emphasis added**

Vitamin D deficiency is not benign. It has devastating consequences. It exists, not in the few, but in the many. Sadly, the epidemic continues.

In this book we will focus on the impact vitamin D deficiency has on the lives of people like you and people like me. For the layperson, this book will provide a unique opportunity to listen to what the scientists are saying about this essential vitamin, all brought down to a level that is easy to understand. This book is also for the physician. For the physician, it will be a great little review of this important topic and exciting area of research.

So, what's all the fuss about a simple vitamin? Good question. What is generally not understood is that this vitamin is not really a vitamin at all! (Holick, 2002; DeLuca, 2004) In its active form, it is a **powerful steroid hormone** (Hollis and Wagner, 2006), considered to be *"one of the most potent hormones for regulating growth."* (Holick, 2006) And the story of this vitamin, this hormone, is quite a story! I will tell it to you in the pages of this book.

Basically, vitamin D is a hormone generated by the skin in response to sunlight then sent on its way to become utilized by the cells to perform any number of very important tasks. Yes, we can ingest this hormone, like we ingest other hormones given to us by prescription, but it is not generally found in significant amounts in our food supply (Decula, 2004). You simply can't get enough vitamin D from an ordinary diet (Holick, 2004b), one that is low in walrus blubber and mackerel (both rich sources of vitamin D, but not usually on the menu). In humans, the skin should be making this hormone for us in plentiful supply, but our modern society has other plans, plans that do not include adequate exposure to sunlight.

There is, however, a Plan B—a very good Plan B! You can take this hormone orally, and do so by eating certain foods or by dietary supplementation. And why would you want this hormone to be in adequate supply? Because there are doctors you just do _not_ want to meet! Doctors who call themselves *Oncologists*; doctors who call themselves *Rheumatologists*; and doctors who call themselves *Endocrinologists*—you don't want to meet these guys! (There are others you will want to stay away from, too, if you can.) These are the very doctors your primary physician is trying his or her best to keep you from becoming well acquainted with. But this may be wishful thinking. Should your physician not be up to speed on the issues related to vitamin D deficiency, or pay little attention to vitamin D in his or her everyday clinical practice, your physician will fail at this task. I see trouble ahead. You will not be served well by any degree of indifference to the hormone we inappropriately call a vitamin. To find out why I can say this in all honesty, you should keep reading.

So let's continue, but only with the understanding that what we are talking about here is *not* a simple vitamin, a simple vitamin that will prevent a simple disease (or two). We are talking about a hormone essential to cellular health and cellular performance. And you won't believe all the trouble you can get into when this hormone is in short supply. Later, you will.

"In this book I will reference just about everything." (The Author, 2014) I don't want you to think that I pulled this stuff out of thin air. And should you share it with your physician (please do), he or she will recognize that what I present is from reputable sources. I will quote the words of physicians and scientists, the ones paying special attention to this area of research. I want you to hear directly from them. In medicine, it's kinda trendy right now to be paying more attention to vitamin D. But soon you will see that, overall, only a little attention is actually being paid, not at all the attention this hormone deserves. And all too often it is simply ignored, as if we do not know what we have here. **Perhaps one of the greatest gifts medical science has to offer us today is the knowledge of what we can accomplish should we start paying close attention to the vitamin that is really a hormone.**

Don't worry; if anything in this book sounds too scientific, it won't when I get done with it! As promised, I will bring the science down to earth and make this as easy on you, the layperson, as I possibly can. You are probably not used to reading medical journals—not when *Gilligan's Island* reruns are so inviting! Therefore, I will try my best to explain in easy-to-understand terms what this hormone is and what this hormone does. If you find a quotation a little difficult to understand, do not despair, things will become clear in the narrative that follows. Although I will use a little humor here (I just can't resist), this is serious business. Come with me and discover what this powerful *hormone* is all about. We will cover a lot of ground here, but it should only take about an hour. Okay, perhaps a little longer, but this will be time well spent.

Perhaps I should mention the reason why this book is written in a somewhat unusual style—all the bold letters and the underlining, and all the other sophisticated writing techniques, all crammed into this little book. You probably won't need a highlighter here! If something is in bold type or italicized, it is undoubtedly very important, I am raising my voice, or I am just getting a little carried away. Should one have a question about the validity of a particular point, a reference will probably be close at hand, built right into the text. The references may seem, at first, to be a little in the way, but soon you will learn to read right past them like they're not even there. And, please, do not skip ahead in the book. Read it straight through or you will miss some of the humor (which would, in itself, be somewhat of a tragedy), fail to grasp certain foundational concepts useful later in the book, and lose some of the momentum that I have skillfully built into this *very* sophisticated presentation. Oh you might not see, at first, all the sophistication that I have packed into this presentation, but let me assure you, it's there. It may be so well hidden, you might not even notice.

Just to be extra nice, I will include a lot of additional stuff, all neatly packed into the little (and not so little) gray boxes that appear at the end of each chapter. This should be fun! (I'll make it fun.)

Behold the gray box!

I love these gray boxes! I use them in all my books. Each gray box I add to the end of a chapter gives me an additional opportunity to discuss with you other things that I feel will contribute significantly to the subject matter at hand. The gray box will become particularly useful should one want to study a particular subject in depth. But they also give me an opportunity to have a little more fun. And we all know how boring medically related books can be. I will change this, one gray box at a time. I *will* be famous for my gray boxes, I just know it.

Chapter 1
Vitamin D: A natural history

Vitamin D is one of the oldest hormones that have been made in the earliest life forms for over 750 million years.

In terms of human history, humans were not confronted with vitamin D deficiency until the industrial revolution began. **~Holick, 2003**

Calling vitamin D a "vitamin" is something of a misnomer. Although the name is still used for historical reasons, vitamin D is more properly classified as a secosteroid because it consists of a cholesterol backbone and exerts steroid-like effects throughout the body, directly affecting the expression of over 1000 genes through the nuclear vitamin D receptor **~Cekic et al., 2011**

Although I am normally compelled to reference just about everything I write (or no one will believe me), in this first chapter I will forgo the references, as the basics of vitamin D are so well established. But later, as we get down to business, I will reference *everything*. So without further ado . . .

Vitamin D has been around for a very long time; it was perhaps the first true hormone in continuous use on planet earth. And it was free, freely derived from the sun. The single-celled creature created it for personal use in many of its metabolic activities. Then along came a hungry multi-celled creature that ate the single-celled creature. And, driven by the need of some creatures to eat other creatures in order to survive, vitamin D became a hormone that could be passed along from creature to creature within the food chain, a hormone useful to the metabolic processes of the one who has not yet been eaten.

Somewhere along the way, along came the hungry human. As luck would have it, the human saw a fish. And so the human ate the fish that ate other little fishes that ate the multi-celled creatures that ate the single-celled creatures. In this manner the human was able to obtain an important ingredient, a hormone if you will, that somehow became necessary to sustain life. But the food chain was just one way to get this hormone. Nudity was another. So, like many other creatures both big and small (and naked), humans were able to obtain vitamin D in abundance by exposure to the sun. Eventually, nudity gave way to clothing (thank god!), and still mankind was able to get plenty of vitamin D, by both diet and sunlight exposure.

So, for what seems like forever, the human race obtained plenty of vitamin D to meet its needs. Then came the industrial revolution, and boy did we get into trouble. And then came the dermatologists with truckloads of sunscreen, and boy did we get into even more trouble.

In the context of reduced exposure to sunlight and changes in diet, humanity is now faced with a host of diseases that are related, in part, to the lack of vitamin D; related, in part, to an immune system that is compromised; related, in part, to a medical profession that just can't seem to wrap its mind around this simple truth: Vitamin D *must* be in adequate supply or people will show up in droves to get drugs to treat diseases that are related, in part, to vitamin D deficiency. Multitudes will suffer. Many will die. That is why I wrote a certain little book about vitamin D.

How vitamin D became so essential to our musculoskeletal system, to our nervous system, to our immune system, even to the hair we grow on our head, is indeed somewhat of a mystery. Many a physician is still waiting for all the details to be worked out before venturing forth and paying very close attention to this vitamin, this hormone, the one we call vitamin D. Fortunately, things are beginning to change. But, be aware, your physician may not be all that into vitamin D, in addition to all the other things he or she is not all that into. I am speaking in generalities, of course. Let's hope that your physician is very knowledgeable in the issues that surround vitamin D and its relationship to the diseases that he or she sees each and every day. But you are clueless, probably, so I will need to get you up to speed.

Let's start with the skin. The skin is really dead. It is the under-the-skin skin that is important to our discussion. Here we find living tissue containing all sorts of things, including cholesterol. As with so many other hormones, cholesterol is the backbone of the vitamin D molecule. Sunlight, specifically the UVB wavelength, has the capacity to displace an electron from the cholesterol molecule, and a hormone is born. This altered cholesterol molecule no longer "fits in" with its neighbors (it must look kinda different) so it is forcibly evicted and eventually finds its way to the liver where it is stored, processed, and sent forth as a prohormone to the kidney or to one of many other organs, tissues, and cells where it is converted by an enzyme called *1-alpha-hydroxylase* into its active form. While in its active form, called *calcitriol* or *1,25(OH)$_2$D$_3$*, vitamin D joins up with a receptor called the VDR and the magic happens. Up to 1000 genes or more can respond, orchestrating genetic events that promote health and resistance to disease. End of story.

So now you know the natural history of vitamin D. As we continue, keep in mind that vitamin D is actually a hormone, a vital hormone. Please keep in mind that you, too, have a natural history, one that is currently in progress. Let's try to make it a lengthy one, one that is a relatively smooth ride. This book should help.

Help me, Dr. Oz, help me!

Since just about everyone is turning to Dr. Oz for advice these days, why don't we? There is a great little video clip on YouTube featuring Dr. Oz on the subject of vitamin D. It includes a nicely prepared animation that demonstrates how vitamin D is manufactured from sunlight. I really want you to see this. Search for:

—**Dr. Oz on The Importance of Vitamin D**
  www.youtube.com/watch?v=6D9aANoN0-Y

Chapter 2
The basics (briefly)

Vitamin D was discovered more than a century ago as the nutrient that prevented rickets, a devastating skeletal disease characterized by under-mineralization of bones. Since that time, our concept of vitamin D . . . has evolved from that of an essential micronutrient to that of a hormone involved in a complex endocrine system that directs mineral homeostasis [regulated balance], protects skeletal integrity, and modulates cell growth and differentiation [advancement into the final form] in a diverse array of tissues. **~Sutton and MacDonald, 2003**

We know that vitamin D is also involved in many nonclassical processes. Vitamin D is devoid of biological activity, but enzymatic conversion to 1α,25-dihydroxyvitamin D [1,25(OH)$_2$D] generates the hormonal form with diverse biological activity. **~Shin et al., 2010**

Vitamin D receptors are common in most tissues in the body, and the new revelation that many tissues produce 1,25-dihydroxy-vitamin D suggests a new important role for this hormone in helping to maintain good health throughout life. **~Holick, 2002**

L et's get this chapter out of the way, and do so without delay—it's beginning to sound a little too scientific for the both of us! But we do need to learn a few basic principles before we continue—you want all of this stuff to make sense, right? This will not be as hard as you think—practically *anything* scientific can be brought down to a level that the layperson can understand. This, of course, is where I come in.

So what is vitamin D? Vitamin D is cholesterol. That's it! Now we can move on. . . . Well, we better learn just a bit more. As mentioned in the preceding chapter, vitamin D is a cholesterol molecule normally found in the deeper layer of the skin, and upon exposure to UVB sunlight, literally becomes bent out of shape, is forcibly ejected from its original location, eventually finds its way to the liver for modification, and finally enters the bloodstream where it circulates to meet the needs of the cells (Holick, 2004a). We must really need this hormone in a big way, because it is *so* easy to make, even for the elderly! (Holick, 2004a; Holick, 2008) Later, the basic vitamin D molecule will be modified by the kidney or a target cell in order to further change it into its active form, a form that the cells can readily put to use. One thing to keep in mind: Vitamin D has several names, and each name depends on the current state of metabolism the cholesterol molecule finds itself in. Also keep in mind that your vitamin D supplement will need to be altered (metabolized) before it can hope to meet the needs of the cells.

Since vitamin D is a hormone, a *very potent hormone,* there are careful controls in place to regulate the availability of its active form. The parathyroid—a collection of four small glands residing next to the thyroid—regulates the circulating level of this "active" vitamin D hormone to within very close tolerances (Sutton and MacDonald, 2003; Holick 2004a; Cui and Rohan, 2006; Holick, 2007) in order to keep the calcium levels within a suitable range so you can continue to live, even when you are, overall, vitamin D deficient (Heaney, 2003). That is why you can have a normal calcium level, a normal parathyroid hormone (PTH) level, even a normal blood level of the active vitamin D hormone, and yet be in a lot of trouble due to a low vitamin D state (Holick, 2002; Holick, 2004b; Sato et al., 2001). This has fooled many a physician in the past (Heaney, 2003; Holick, 2004a; Steingrimsdottir et al., 2005). Perhaps it still does. A normal calcium level, sometimes looked at to determine if a patient is vitamin D sufficient, can mislead the unsuspecting physician into thinking that the vitamin D status of the patient *must* be satisfactory (Holick, 2004a). If **you** are this patient, one with a low vitamin status that persists, a slow, imperceptible deterioration of your skeletal system may result—even when your calcium intake is normal.

When vitamin D levels are low, less calcium is absorbed through the small intestine (Holick, 2002), perhaps not enough to meet the overall needs of the body. Attention is then directed at the skeletal system— "Hey, let's take some calcium from the bones. They have so much, and they'll never miss it! Besides, we promise to pay it back." If you've heard of *osteoporosis*, what you've heard of is a broken promise—and you may not know the price you have paid until you fall and break a hip. But all this borrowing has occurred for a higher purpose. The bones have been called upon to meet the calcium needs of the rest of the body (DeLuca, 2004; Heaney, 2003; Holick, 2002). This consistent "borrowing" (and *never* paying back) can go on for up to 10 years before structural damage becomes clinically evident (Heaney, 2003). It is not by accident; it is good intention, at least in part, that leads to the disease we call osteoporosis. Even when large amounts of calcium are taken in an effort to reduce the risk of osteoporosis, or to slow its progression, success will be limited in the setting of low vitamin D availability. Certainly other factors are involved, but make no mistake; vitamin D deficiency will have a negative impact on the integrity of skeletal system, perhaps <u>your</u> skeletal system. I see trouble ahead.

In a low vitamin D state, the small intestine can absorb approximately 10% to 15% of dietary calcium. When vitamin D levels are adequate, intestinal absorption of dietary calcium more than doubles, rising to approximately 30% to 40%. Thus, when vitamin D levels (25[OH]D) are low, calcium absorption is insufficient to satisfy the calcium requirements not only for bone health but also for most metabolic functions and neuromuscular activity. (Holick, 2006a)

We'll talk more about calcium later (and perhaps a little more about vitamin D), but keep this in mind: Life is calcium in action. Nerve function is dependent on calcium availability (McCann and Ames, 2008). Muscle strength and function, too, relies on calcium availability (Holick, 2002). And other cells, too, require calcium in order to maintain their very existence and perform many of their essential tasks (Heaney, 2003;

Peterlik and Cross, 2005; Holick, 2006b). At the cellular level, vitamin D is involved not only in calcium regulation within the cell (Zittermann, 2003) but also in a myriad of other cellular events that keep us functioning as intended (Holick, 2004b; VanAmerongen et al., 2004). Everywhere, calcium and vitamin D work together, hand in hand (Chi and Rohan, 2006). But as prominent as the relationship between calcium and vitamin D is, let's not forget about the kidney. The kidney plays a very important role in the story of vitamin D.

The kidney will take the vitamin D produced by the skin (or ingested) and create a baseline level of the active hormone in the bloodstream for use by tissues and cells. This active hormone is called $1,25(OH)_2D_3$, basically because it needed some kind of fancy name. Another name for this active form of vitamin D is *Calcitriol*. But it is still cholesterol! It has just had a makeover and received a name change.

Now in order to generate enough of the active form of this hormone at the cellular level, the cells themselves, not relying solely upon what the kidney will produce, will modify the vitamin D formation that is processed by the liver, $(25(OH)D_3)$, and turn it into $1,25(OH)_2D_3$. Of course this all depends on availability (Lappe et al., 2007) and the activity of certain enzymes that make it all possible. What is surprising is that we were able to cure the devastating disease called rickets— **regarded as one of the greatest triumphs in medical history** (DeLuca, 2004)—long before we had a clue that it was this "active" form of vitamin D that was doing the trick. Not so great was the idea that the dose of vitamin D needed to prevent or cure rickets was the same dose needed to maintain overall health and to protect us from a variety of other diseases—**big mistake!** Decades later, we are still paying the price for this unfortunate misunderstanding. (see Heaney, 2003; Holick, 2006b; Vieth, 1999)

What was not known in the days of curing rickets left and right was that this hormone is *"involved in countless physiological functions"* (VanAmerongen et al., 2004) involving more than **50** different tissues (McCann and Ames, 2008). You probably do not think of yourself as a collection of tissues, but you are! And almost every tissue or cell type that forms **you** needs vitamin D (Holick, 2005). This is a hormone that triggers, or stops, or in some way regulates—even by joining forces with other hormones (Spina et al., 2006)—upwards of 1,000 genes and associated genetic events (Holick, 2006a; Ginde et al., 2009), perhaps more! **Vitamin D is a regulator of genes. That is what it does. In this manner, it regulates the actions and the performance of cells.** We did not know this back in the days of curing rickets left and right. And some observers might question if we act like we know it today. Even today, not enough attention is being paid to the hormone we call a vitamin. As we continue, you will see how tragic this really is.

When a gene is improperly regulated, problems occur. We go to the doctor (often repeatedly) for problems related to the improper regulation of genetic events. When a hormone regulates a gene, it should be in adequate supply (Wagoner et al., 2008). If the hormone is not in adequate supply, the cell will face challenges, challenges that it should not have to face. There are, however, genetic programs that seem to help us compensate for low vitamin D availability (many associated cellular events are downregulated or silenced in the face of low substrate availability) so the individual can squeak by.

The message of this chapter is simple: Vitamin D is a vital regulator of many genetic events—important genetic events. The genetic event may be the creation of a protein that will be bravely sent on its way, all the way from one location in a cell to another location way over there in some remote part of the same cell—all to keep things running smoothly, of course. (To a little molecule, a cell is a *very* big thing!) The genetic event may even be the creation of a molecule that, too, will be bravely sent on its way to another cell in order to influence the level of activity and/or the behavior of the target cell. The genetic event may even be the synthesis of a molecule needed to keep your nervous system running smoothly so that depression does not set in (Miller, 2007). But there is even more to the story. Some cells, following insult and injury, actually signal other cells to begin various stages of healing and repair. This is particularly true with respect to the inflammatory response. Inflammation, a well-coordinated activity at the cellular level, intended to resolve a problem and set the stage for resolution and healing, is regulated, in part, by vitamin D (Schwartz, 2002; Whitton, 2007; Adorini and Penna, 2008; VanAmerongen et al., 2004). Even healing itself is regulated by vitamin D (Adorini and Penna, 2008). So the *successful* regulation of genetic events is undoubtedly one very important matter.

What the cell does, what the cell is, stems from unbelievably complex programs stored within the cell nucleus, or stored in the mitochondria that inhabit the cell. Accordingly, vitamin D works its magic—not only at the nuclear level (Spina et al., 2006) but also at the level of the mitochondria, the energy-producing factories of the cell (Eyles et al., 2007). Just to underscore how complex all of this is, a cell, so small that it cannot be seen by the naked eye, may hold as many as 10,000 mitochondria all packed in there somewhere! Each one has its own set of genes, is mobile within the cell, and has a variety of important tasks to perform. And each one needs vitamin D. **Vitamin D replacement, therefore, is therapy for genes, genes that regulate the maintenance of health and well-being.** Your risk of disease—and there are *so many* diseases to choose from—is elevated when vitamin D is not in adequate supply.

Let's take a short break (after the grey box below) and continue with the basics of vitamin D in the following chapter.

Would you like to see mitochondria in action?

You're nodding "yes," aren't you? Well, do I have a *great* little video for you! As you view this video, and marvel, keep in mind that your life as we know it is totally dependent on what you are watching. Keep this in mind, too: Mitochondria play a big role the vitamin D story.

Mitochondria are the energy producers of the cell, generating a cellular fuel called ATP. All cells have them. Some have only one or two (like the silly illustration in your old biology book). But for most cells one or two mitochondria per cell simply does not cut it, not even close. For example: The muscle of a well-trained athlete may have as many as

4,000 mitochondria, *per cell!* And if that's not impressive enough: The cells of the eye responsible for vision—a high-energy process—may contain as many as 10,000 mitochondria per cell. This is truly amazing! So have a little fun, log on to YouTube, and watch:

—Powering the Cell: Mitochondria
www.youtube.com/watch?v=RrS2uROUjK4

One reason I want you to watch this video is the fact that vitamin D (magically, sort of) finds its way to the mitochondria, is incorporated into many of its activities, and is involved in the creation of the energy the cell will need to survive and to thrive. Important to our conversation, vitamin D deficiency lowers energy production within the cell, and the cell may simply squeak by and live a life of compromise. Surprisingly, molecular motors, such as shown in the featured video— shown rotating in slow motion—may rotate at a speed of 42,000 revolutions per minute! (Nakanishi-Matsui et al., 2006) And I've seen reports as high as 96,000 RPM! I am blown away by the mitochondria! I am blown away by molecular motors! I am blown away by this video! However, I am not blown away by you. I consider you to be a challenge at this point in time. Regardless, I will be a little more impressed with you if you can accomplish the following . . .

Can you solve this mystery?

In the 1920s, a time when scientists were trying to understand why both sunlight and cod liver oil not only prevented but also cured rickets, a little mystery popped up, unexpectedly. The scientists were stumped, as is so often the case. I will share with you this fascinating story, and it goes something like this:

Rickets baffled medicine for centuries. A home remedy, cod liver oil, seemed to be the cure. But why? Sunlight was known to both prevent and cure this devastating disease. But why? No one knew why. So the scientists set out to find out. To make a long story short, a particular series of experiments was conducted, arising from a very unusual accidental finding during the study of rats with experimental rickets.

Science, at this time in history, knew all about UVB radiation, a portion of the invisible light spectrum that caused certain biological effects to occur. In fact, they had been using UVB irradiation of food to create a bioactive "something," later to be identified and called vitamin D. If UVB could create this "something" in food—and a rat is, of course, food—why not, using UVB radiation, irradiate rats that have rickets just to see what would happen? As anticipated, after treatment the rats were cured of rickets, and great joy was felt both in the laboratory and throughout the land. But to the surprise of the scientists, all they had to do was irradiate the inside of the jar that the rats were housed in, with the rats kept elsewhere, and the rats would recover soon after they were returned to the irradiated jar. *This* was indeed a mystery! Why were the returning rats cured of rickets? And so it came to pass, another series of experiments were conducted in order to figure out what exactly was taking place. Of course, this was a confusing time for the rats, but little thought was given to that because they were, after all, just rats. Have you figured it out yet? Have you solved the mystery? Hint: If you take a *cured* rat from the irradiated jar and put it in with other rats that had rickets, the diseased rats, too, would be cured of the disease.

The answer to the mystery is quite a surprise. It was the skin oil on the fur of the irradiated rat, converted to vitamin D upon exposure to UVB radiation and then deposited on the inside of the empty jar, that provided enough vitamin D for all. So, all you have to do, as a rat, is to rub up against the inside of your enclosure, rub up against your roommates, groom yourself and your roommate and the roommate of your roommate, and you could easily satisfy your vitamin D requirements and help others do the same. I suppose, in order to save a little money, you could get involved in all the grooming and such, but I would not recommend it, and others may not quite understand. Why go to all the bother, say I, when vitamin D is *so easy* to obtain by sunlight exposure or by taking vitamin D in capsule form.

This story is told in the following paper:

—**Carpenter KJ, Zhao L** 1999 Forgotten Mysteries in the Early History of Vitamin D. J. Nutr. 129:923–927

Chapter 3
Action at the nuclear level (sorry, more science)

Vitamin D . . . modulates cell growth and differentiation in a diverse array of tissues.   **~Sutton and MacDonald, 2003**

The vitamin D hormone system controls the expression of more than 200 genes and the proteins they produce. In addition to its well known role in calcium metabolism, vitamin D activates genes that control cell growth and programmed cell death (apoptosis), express mediators that regulate the immune system, and release neurotransmitters (e.g., serotonin) that influence one's mental state.   **~Miller, 2007**

The VDR receptor has been identified in almost every tissue and cell including brain, heart, skin, pancreas, breast, colon, and immune cells. **~Holick, 2005**

One of the most intriguing important and unappreciated biological functions of $1,25(OH)_2D$ is its ability to down-regulate hyperproliferative (excessive) cell growth. Normal and cancer cells that have a vitamin D receptor often respond to $1,25(OH)_2D$ by decreasing their proliferation and enhancing their maturation.   **~Holick, 2004a**

High calcium intakes reduce circulating concentrations of calcitriol [the "active" vitamin D], which in turn, is known to shorten the half-life of serum 25(OH)D—i.e., higher calcium concentrations result in <u>greater metabolic consumption and degradation</u> of 25(OH)D, effectively lowering vitamin D status.   **~Lappe et al., 2007, emphasis added**

In the previous chapter, I made reference to the fact that the actions of vitamin D occur basically within the cell, particularly at the level of the cell nucleus. Interestingly, the conversion of *pre*-vitamin D into *active*-vitamin D, when it occurs in the kidney, occurs within the mitochondria that inhabit the kidney cell (Holick, 2006). But there is a whole lot more to the story. We need a little more science under our belt before we get too far along in this presentation. I'm making this stuff easy, right?

First, there is this thing called a *VDR*, short for *Vitamin D Receptor*. A VDR is a cellular formation that is mobile within the cell (VanAmerongen, 2004), interacts with a vitamin D molecule once it arrives, changes in form, invites other molecules (coactivators) to get involved in the action, and is then guided (actually dragged) along what are called microtubules to the nucleus or a mitochondria by what are called *motor proteins* (Kamimura et al., 1995). (I call them delivery proteins.) Once the vitamin D/VDR complex reaches the nucleus, for example, it is actively transported within (Holick, 2004b; Spina et al., 2006), to the place where the genetic-event-business really transpires (VanAmerongen et al., 2004; Holick, 2004b).

Second—and this is a surprise—you can actually make your vitamin D status worse by trying to do yourself a favor (or so you think). I'll explain shortly, but first, more about the VDR.

The VDR is a protein formation found within the cell, a formation that is itself, no doubt, created by genetic programs found therein. The role of the VDR is to bind the active form of vitamin D and become available for transport into the cell nucleus in order to target and <u>directly</u> stimulate the activity of upwards of 200 genes. Indirectly, the vitamin D/VDR complex may work in concert with other hormones and other factors and thereby influence up to 1,000 genes, perhaps more! I'll bet more than a few of those genes are involved in keeping you from falling apart at the seams—that's how important certain genes are! This is why the cell makes somewhere between **100,000 to 1,000,000** repairs to its DNA, per day, per cell! (source: Wikipedia, 2010) (I'm blown away again!) For certain, some genes keep you from getting cancer, some genes keep you from being attacked by your own immune cells, and some genes keep your nervous system from going nuts (medical term).

Now for the surprise: As we get older, our bones just seem to want to fall apart (we know what happened to Grandma). Osteoporosis is a very concerning medical problem, is the focus of much attention, and certainly needs to be addressed, its progress halted and reversed. I've mentioned this before. Eventually, you and your physician will need to sit down to decide just what to do next. And I know how this conversation is going to turn out. You will no doubt be increasing your calcium intake. But this, *by itself*, is simply not enough. It may even be harmful. Let me explain:

If your low vitamin D status is not identified and not *sufficiently* addressed (i.e., you are maintained in a relatively vitamin D-deficient state), you could be increasing your risk of heart disease while you are trying your best to prevent osteoporosis (Bollan et al., 2010). Read again the last quotation at the beginning of this chapter. (You read it carefully, right?) **By attempting to improve your bone density just by taking extra calcium, you will be taking resources away from other cellular processes that are also dependent on an adequate supply of vitamin D.** Processes like the ones that keep you from getting cancer, that keep your immune system well regulated, and that keep you from becoming depressed (Wagner et al., 2008). **A high calcium intake without a sufficient intake of vitamin D will lower your overall vitamin D status** (Vieth, 1999; Lappe et al., 2007; VanAmerongen et al., 2004). I see trouble ahead. The extra vitamin D that may be added to the calcium supplement may be somewhat helpful, but it is simply not enough to make a major difference. I, personally, would *insist* on having a vitamin D level drawn and insist on having this issue *appropriately* addressed before embarking on an increased calcium regimen. *"Unless a 25 (OH)D level is determined, it is impossible to know if a person is sufficient in vitamin D. Further, symptoms of vitamin D deficiency are very subtle and often go undetected."* (Holick, 2002) Clearly, increasing calcium intake should be done in concert with the identification and correction of a low vitamin D state (Cui and Rohan, 2006). You need sufficiency in both.

In case you were in a hurry (to see what Gilligan is up to now) and did not go back and re-read the quote that I asked you to read, I'll give you another opportunity. It's that important! So important, in fact, that I will repeat it and place it in bold letters. I am that nice.

> **High calcium intakes reduce circulating concentrations of calcitriol [the active vitamin D], which in turn, is known to shorten the half-life of serum 25(OH)D—i.e., higher calcium concentrations result in greater metabolic consumption and degradation of 25(OH)D, effectively lowering vitamin D status.** (Lappe et al., 2007, emphasis added to get your attention)

I have one more statement to share, one that will help emphasize the importance of adequate vitamin D supplementation in your quest to prevent osteoporosis by calcium supplementation. This statement, too, is important enough to warrant bold lettering.

> **Calcium supplements (without coadminstration with vitamin D) are associated with an increased risk of myocardial infarction.** (Bolland et al., 2010, emphasis added)

So now that you have the basics of vitamin D under your belt (and you are trembling a bit), we can continue. In the pages to follow, I will share with you the impact vitamin D deficiency has on the lives of people like you and people like me. But before I forget, may I ask you this?

What actually happened to Grandma?

Life is particularly hard if you bear this title. But does it have to be? Could vitamin D prevent at least some of the wear and tear that goes into the making of a grandma? The answer is, convincingly, *yes*.

Any grandma that I am aware of started off as something else, and most got their start in life at a time when little attention was paid to vitamin D. As a result, some potential grandmas never had the opportunity to get beyond childhood, and many never made it that far. Throughout history, rickets has taken so many lives during birth, of both mother and child, that it simply boggles the mind. Something as simple as adequate sunlight or adequate intake of vitamin D could have prevented so much loss and so much anguish, and not that long ago. Even in the early 1900s many mothers died during childbirth simply because their pelvic architecture was deformed and insufficient to allow for fetal passage—easily preventable by vitamin D sufficiency. Fortunately, your grandma survived all of this. But there were other challenges in store.

Without adequate exposure to sunlight, because one cannot typically get enough vitamin D by normal dietary practices, Grandma was at great risk for a variety of medical conditions as she progressed through the aging process. Her risk of infections, both common and life-threatening, was increased. Her risk of hormonal imbalance was increased, and hormonal imbalance no doubt occurred—and Grandpa got hollered at a lot, and for little or no reason. Her risk of cancer, heart disease, autoimmune disorders, depression, toothlessness, and so on, also became increased by vitamin D deficiency. It's tough being a grandma, and our society seems to make it tougher. Even the clothes dryer, invented to make her life easier, was out to kill her, preventing her from going outside in all that beautiful, vitamin D–producing sunshine to hang clothes out on the clothesline. I will venture a guess, your grandma lived a vitamin D-deficient life and suffered from many diseases that, perhaps, could have been easily prevented or lessened in severity by vitamin D sufficiency.

So, many things happened to Grandma along the way, and falling and breaking a hip makes the impact of vitamin D deficiency so painfully apparent. I hope this never happens to you. But it certainly could have happened to your grandma. As a recovery room nurse, every day, or so it seems, I take care of an individual (a grandma) who has recently fallen and can't get up, having suffered a fractured hip. Even today, grandmas (and grandpas) die as a result of a fractured hip, and great sadness is felt throughout the land.

Don't forget the calcium (and the vitamin D)

No, I don't mind drilling this into your head, if that's what it takes. But you may need a little break from me. So why not listen to these guys for a few moments?

The wide range of diseases associated with defects in calcium and vitamin D in combination with the high prevalence of these conditions represents a special challenge for preventative medicine.

Vitamin D or calcium insufficiency, respectively, contribute to the development of chronic diseases by different pathogenic mechanisms (as detailed earlier). A nutritional calcium deficit or a compromised vitamin D status has been identified as an independent risk factor, as in the case of colon cancer. More often, however, the calcium and vitamin D statuses appear to act largely together, such as in the pathogenesis of osteoporosis, colorectal and breast cancer, and probably also of autoimmune diabetes type I and multiple sclerosis.

The fact that, as detailed earlier, almost one quarter of the healthy adult population presents with a compromised vitamin D status and, at the same time appears also to be calcium deficient, poses a special challenge for preventative medicine and public health policy alike. (Peterlik and Cross, 2005, emphasis added)

Improving calcium and vitamin D nutritional status substantially reduces all-cancer risk in postmenopausal women. (Lappe et al., 2007, emphasis added)

Vitamin D is essential for the efficient unitization of dietary calcium. (Holick, 2003)

Chapter 4
Let's face it, you're not getting enough!

According to several studies, 40 to 100% of U.S. and European elderly men and women still living in the community (not in nursing homes) are deficient in vitamin D. ~**Holick, 2007**

Vitamin D deficiency has been reported in approximately 36% of otherwise healthy young adults and up to 57% of general medicine inpatients in the United States and in even higher percentages in Europe. ~**Holick, 2006a**

Ironically, the sun is all around us, yet so are the diseases that are related to a lack of sufficient sunlight exposure—and the list is indeed a long one. Something is clearly wrong with this picture. In your case, *you* may be the problem. Just look at your lifestyle and you will see how easy it is to become and remain deficient in vitamin D. I am assuming, for the moment, that you are a gentleman. For you ladies, I'll write you in here somewhere.

You probably wake up early each weekday morning, eat a sensible breakfast, *never* forget to kiss the wife goodbye, and get in the car and drive to work behind steel and glass at the time of day that will not allow you to generate vitamin D from sunlight no matter how hard you try. Creating vitamin D in a significant amount requires exposure to sunlight between the hours of 10 AM and 3 PM (Holick, 2004)—perhaps as late as 6 PM in certain geographical regions (Holick, 2006b). From around October to March, you might as well forget it!—the sun travels across the sky at too low of an angle to allow any appreciable amount of UVB radiation to penetrate the atmosphere (VanAmerongen et al., 2004), that is unless you live high up in the Alps (or elsewhere) where a thinner atmosphere allows more UVB radiation to penetrate (Hayes et al., 1997). During winter, you will need to rely exclusively on vitamin D supplementation (diet or otherwise) and on your fat stores of vitamin D. Good thing you had a glass of vitamin D-fortified orange juice this morning; but, in order to compensate for insufficient UVB exposure, you should have drunked, dranken, drinked—let's just say "consumed" 20 glasses of orange juice this morning! Who has that kind of time? And this is one of your typical days! Fortunately, however, the weekend has rolled around and now you're in luck!

We know what the weekend means! It is now time to mow the lawn (as long as it doesn't interfere with watching the game). And I know that you will be doing the honors, because you, like me, are basically too cheap to pay the neighbor boy to do it for you. Now is your chance to get upwards of 20,000 units of vitamin D in one fell swoop (Holick, 2002; Wagner et al., 2008), if the sun is shining, your lawn is big enough, and you mow the lawn . . . *naked?!!* (You learned this from the internet, didn't you?) Perhaps this level of sunlight exposure will help get you through the next several days. Oh! You can take comfort in the fact that the wife is probably satisfying her need for vitamin D, too. While you are mowing the lawn naked, in a well-meaning but somewhat misguided effort to absorb more sunlight, she is walking down to the river to bathe. On the way back home, she will probably spend a little extra time in the sun, gathering sticks for a fire over which she will cook the evening meal (provided that you are a good hunter-gatherer and you have made a fresh kill—hopefully not with your lawn mower!). You make a fine couple for the neighbors to stare at and seriously consider moving far away from. I, however, would find both you and your wife quite entertaining and would want to keep you around, just for fun.

What is clearly wrong with our lifestyle today is that we are not generating enough vitamin D in the intended way. Adequate, consistent sunlight exposure is clearly Plan A. And Plan B, it's just not working! When you look at the new recommendations for vitamin D levels and the statistics on vitamin D deficiency, there seem to be more vitamin D-deficient people on the planet than there are people on the planet! Wait! I'm not quite sure about this statistic. I'll be back in a few minutes.

Okay, I'm back! Well, I may have overestimated the problem just a little. I now have some more realistic statistics to share with you—but they are probably not all that accurate either. Why? We are just beginning to realize that the new "normal" level of vitamin D is more than twice as high as it was just a few years ago. And what was an acceptable level in the not-too-distant past may be 3 or 4 times too low according to the latest research (Spina et al., 2006). So, as the recommended levels are revised upwardly, statistics will change. For me, it takes 8,000 IU per day to keep my vitamin D level within the latest recommendations (I cut back on the days that I get extra sun exposure). Be that as it may, let's take a look at a few statistics that have recently been published:

- "It has been estimated that **1 billion** people worldwide have vitamin D deficiency or insufficiency." (Holick, 2007, emphasis added)

- "It was recently shown that only **4%** of adults ≥ 51 years old consume the recommended AI [adequate intake]." (Spina et al., 2006, emphasis added

- "**Almost one quarter** of the healthy adult population presents with a compromised vitamin D status and, at the same time appears also to be calcium deficient . . . ." (Peterlik and Cross, 2005, emphasis added

- "It is estimated that **> 50%** of African Americans in the United States are either chronically or seasonally at risk of vitamin D deficiency." (Holick, 2004, emphasis added)

- "A study of Asian adults in the United Kingdom showed that **82%** had 25(OH)D levels less than 12 ng/ml (30 nmol/L) during the summer season, with the proportion increasing to **94%** during the winter months." (Holick, 2006a, emphasis added)

- "A rapidly evolving knowledge base indicates that vitamin D deficiency is much more prevalent than previously recognized and is present in up to **50%** of young adults and children." (Lee et al., 2008, emphasis added)

You do <u>not</u> want to know the statistics on infants and the newborn—way too disturbing! Suffice it to say, a vitamin D-deficient mother will *not* pass vitamin D on to her nursing infant as intended. (see Wagner et al., 2008 for review) That is, unless the nursing infant is getting adequate supplementation, is receiving a vitamin D-sufficient formula, or is fortunate enough to have one of those combination crib/UVB tanning booths. Without vitamin D sufficiency in the infant, again, I see trouble ahead. Kids these days are just not resistant to infectious diseases (McGrath et al., 2004), not even close. Just wait until they go to school and pick up every "bug" that is suitable for passing on to you! It takes an efficient, well-orchestrated immune system for both children and adults to be infectious-disease resistant. Clearly, vitamin D is a central player in the efficiency and effectiveness of our immune system, but this all depends on availability.

So if vitamin D should be in adequate supply in order to sustain the genetic programs that give us the gift of life, health, and a sense of well-being, just imagine what would happen should vitamin D be in short supply! Cells and biological systems would just not function as effectively as intended. But you don't have to imagine. The consequences are all around us! Just look at the diseases that are associated with *Western Civilization* (the indoor people)—these diseases, they're everywhere!

Have I got a book for you!

Yes, I have another book on vitamin D entitled **Mommy, Me, and Vitamin D**. In it, I focus on the impact vitamin D deficiency has on babies, even mommies, both during gestation and later in life. You won't believe all the damage it does.

> Vitamin D deficiency during pregnancy is the origin of a host of future perils for the child. Some of this damage done by maternal vitamin D deficiency becomes evident after many years. Therefore, prevention of vitamin D deficiency among pregnant women is essential. (Kaushal and Magon, 2013)

Vitamin D deficiency is an open invitation to a whole host of diseases, inviting them to come, find your child, and destroy. Many are lost before birth. Many, later in life, are claimed by type I diabetes, multiple sclerosis, Crohn's disease, and other *"perils"* that harm, destroy futures, and destroy lives. You will treasure this book. It is available on Amazon.com and at my website:

—www.impactofvitamind.com

Chapter 5
Overview: The price we are paying

Vitamin D deficiency is linked to inflammatory and long-latency diseases such as multiple sclerosis, rheumatoid arthritis, tuberculosis, diabetes, and various cancers, to name a few.   **~Wagner et al., 2008, emphasis added**

It is well known that poor 25OHD3 [vitamin D] status is common in many human diseases associated with inflammation, including infection, autoimmune diseases, obesity and metabolic syndrome, type 2 diabetes, osteoporosis, cancer, and cardiovascular diseases.   **~McCann and Ames, 2008, emphasis added**

Hypovitaminosis D [low vitamin D status] is therefore not only a pathogenetic factor for bone diseases such as rickets, osteomalacia and osteoporosis, but also plays an important though <u>largely underestimated</u> role in the development of malignant, chronic inflammatory and autoimmune diseases as well as metabolic disorders.

Compromised vitamin D status in humans increases the risk of Th-1 cytokine-mediated autoimmune disorders, such as inflammatory bowel disease, rheumatoid arthritis, systemic lupus erythematoses, multiple sclerosis as well as type I diabetes mellitus.   **~Peterlik and Cross, 2005, emphasis added**

Mounting evidence indicates a high prevalence of vitamin D deficiency in the general population, and this deficiency has been linked to an increased incidence of autoimmune diseases, as well as bone diseases and cancer.   **~Adorini and Pinna, 2008, emphasis added**

It is now well documented that the risk of developing and dying of colon, prostate, breast, ovarian, esophageal, non-Hodgkin's lymphoma, and a variety of other lethal cancers is related to living at higher latitudes and being more at risk of vitamin D deficiency. **~Holick, 2005, emphasis added**

I just *had* to squeeze some more great quotes in here somewhere, so I came up with this little chapter! And in this chapter, I will write one of the most profound statements you are ever going to read, anywhere! You'll find it in a few moments. I'll be sure to place it in bold letters so you won't miss it.

In our society we have a big problem on our hands, commonly referred to as *vitamin D deficiency*. But, as with any other medical problem, the scientists have made up a fancy name just to make things seem more dreadful. Accordingly, vitamin D deficiency is more formally called *hypovitaminosis D*. Actually it is kinda dreadful, but in a roundabout sort of way. **You don't actually die from hypovitaminosis D itself, it just makes it easier for other things to kill you!** When you read about all the trouble you can get into when vitamin D supplies are inadequate, keep in mind that vitamin D can also help manage and improve the very medical conditions that are brought about by its deficiency—not all the time, but at least a good share of the time. Prevention, of course, is always the best course of action. All would agree, it is better to prevent a dreadful disease than it is to try to deal with all the messiness once a dreadful disease becomes evident and alters a life in unspeakable ways.

The research is clear. The risk of many medical conditions substantially increases when vitamin D status is inadequate to very low, and many diseases have been shown to respond, in a significant way, with vitamin D supplementation. Here are a few examples:

- "In one study, 5,000 IU of vitamin D/d, along with calcium and magnesium supplementation, **reduced exacerbations in MS** [multiple sclerosis] patients by 59% compared with previous year(s)." (VanAmerongen et al., 2004, emphasis added)

- "Normal vitamin D status has been linked to favorable health outcomes ranging from **decreased risk of osteoporosis** to **improved cancer mortality**." (Fakih et al., 2009, emphasis added)

- "McAlindon et al observed that a higher intake of vitamin D and higher blood levels of 25(OH)D **decreased progression of osteoarthritis in men and women by more than 60%.**" (Holick, 2006, emphasis added)

- "Chronic vitamin D deficiency may have serious adverse consequences, including increased risk of hypertension, multiple sclerosis, cancers of the colon, prostate, breast, and ovary, and type 1 diabetes." (Holick, 2003)

As we continue moving through the pages of this book, we'll take a look at the above-mentioned diseases, and others, in order to understand the role vitamin D deficiency may be (probably is) playing in the development of diseases you could certainly live without. We'll begin with cancer, a disease that strikes fear into the hearts of even the brave. And please read each introductory quotation at the beginning of the following chapter very carefully—very important! But first, consider this:

How to talk to your doctor about vitamin D

So, you feel your physician may not be up to speed on vitamin D— have you had a vitamin D level drawn . . . ever? Has your doctor recommended that you be on 400 IU/d, 1,000 IU/d, or at best, 2,000 IU/d of vitamin D without having a clue what your vitamin D level is?

Sure signs that he or she may not be all that cutting-edge when it comes to the issues surrounding vitamin D. So, here is what you do:

1) Place a telephone call to your physician _today_! Pleasantly request a lab draw for a 25(OH)D level. Don't take "No" for an answer! Tell him or her that drawing a vitamin D level now will save time and provide something important to discuss (for a change) during the next office visit. Smile while you speak, everyone responds to a smile.

2) Then, when you _finally_ get in to see the doctor, simply start the conversation by saying, "I know you don't want me to come down with something dreadful like inflammatory bowel disease, rheumatoid arthritis, systemic lupus erythematosis, paracoccidioidomycosis (if you can pronounce this), multiple sclerosis, diabetes, cancer, etc., etc., do you? So what are we going to do about this—this _alarmingly_ low vitamin D level that I'm sure I have come down with?" And, "You don't want me to die of cancer any time soon, do you? **What good am I to you dead?!!**" (These are just examples; you can make up other stuff in order to get the doctor's attention.)

3) Next, after enduring such remarks as **"Calm down!"** and "Have you been reading that _Impact of Vitamin D Deficiency_ book lately?" proceed to explain that you want your vitamin D status _expertly_ managed and that you want to achieve and maintain a _respectable_ vitamin D level. You can mention that you can find another doctor, should the need arise. (Be sure to smile if you feel the need to issue this warning. Everyone responds to a smile.)

The above strategy, or any part thereof, should produce some results. But keep the following in mind: One vitamin D level is just not enough. After you start to correct a low vitamin D status, you need follow-up labs to see if you have accomplished your goal of becoming vitamin D sufficient. They can also indicate if you are getting too much vitamin D. And labs should be taken at least yearly (better, every 3 to 5 days—just kidding!) to see if your vitamin D level is being maintained at an appropriate level. But remember, your physician may have a very good reason not to be aggressive with vitamin D, or not to prescribe it at all! Let me explain:

A few medical conditions actually require an avoidance of supplemental vitamin D, such as sarcoidosis, "active" inflammatory bowel disease, and a certain form of cancer (referenced below). There are a few good reasons to use caution, but not many. Listen closely to what your physician has to say; just don't let your vitamin D status be ignored or treated ineffectively. *Never* be afraid to seek a second opinion.

If you want to read a great paper on vitamin D, one that is written for the physician but is fairly easy for the layperson to follow, I recommend **Not Enough Vitamin D: Health Consequences for Canadians** by Gary Schwalfenberg, MD, CCFP. This paper is available free online and is a great reference to have. (It would also make a fine gift for the physician—they are always looking around for something to read.) On the last page of the article, Dr. Schwalfenberg lists potential side effects of vitamin D supplementation, as well as certain medical conditions where supplemental vitamin D is not advisable, as follows:

> Reported side effects of vitamin D include nausea, vomiting, headache, metallic taste, vascular or nephrocalcinosis, and pancreatitis. Reported contraindications to vitamin D include hypercalcemia in sarcoidosis; metastatic bone disease; other granulomatous diseases such as tuberculosis and Crohn's disease (active phase) that have a disordered vitamin D metabolism in activated macrophages; and Williams syndrome (infantile hypercalcemia). (Schwalfenberg, 2007)

Chapter 6
Cancer

Vitamin D . . . modulates cell growth and differentiation in a diverse array of tissues. **~Sutton and MacDonald, 2003**

A more recent analysis estimated that **currently between 50,000– 63,000 Americans and 19,000–25,000 individuals living in the United Kingdom annually die prematurely from cancer due to vitamin D deficiency.** **~Spina et al., 2006, emphasis added**

The inverse association between ambient solar radiation and cancer mortality rates has subsequently been described for cancers of the breast, rectum, ovary, prostate, stomach, bladder, esophagus, kidney, lung, pancreas, and uterus, as well as for non-Hodgkin lymphoma and multiple myeloma. **~Lappe et al., 2007**

The correlation between decreased morbidity and mortality of cancer and exposure to sunlight is known. The many biological functions of vitamin D that contribute to cancer prevention have only begun to be appreciated. Once activated, 1,25dihydroxyvitamin D [1,25 (OH)$_2$D$_3$] functions as a <u>potent inhibitor</u> *of normal cancer cellular proliferation. Vitamin D deficiency in mice led to a 60% increase in colon tumor growth, compared to vitamin D-sufficient mice.* **~Spina et al., 2006, emphasis added**

The most bioactive form of vitamin D [1,25(OH)$_2$D$_3$] modulates cell proliferation, differentiation, cancer invasion, and angiogenesis [development of a supportive vascular supply]. **~Bläuer et al., 2009**

Since the 1940s, it has been recognized that people who live at higher latitudes have a higher risk of dying of the most common cancers, including colon, breast, and prostate. It is also known that normal adults with a 25(OH)2D3 of at least 20 ng/ml have a 50% decreased risk of developing colon cancer.   **~Holick, 2003**

The report that postmenopausal women who increased their vitamin D intake by 1100 IU of vitamin D₃ reduced their relative risk of cancer by **60 to 77%** *is a compelling reason to be vitamin D-sufficient.*   **~Holick, 2007, emphasis added**

C learly we are at an increased risk of cancer should we live a life deficient in vitamin D. And, of course, nothing grabs our attention like hearing the word "cancer," particularly so when sitting in front of a physician, one who is not smiling at the moment. Tragically, 1 out of 4 individuals walking among us will die from this disease, one individual at a time, unless we do something relevant to prevent it. I have something relevant in mind.

When it comes to cancer, the cell is not thinking things through very carefully—one way or another, it's gonna die! So what is cancer? What is going wrong? And, most importantly, what can be done to prevent it?

Cancer is basically a collection of previously normal cells that have somehow changed, are multiplying rapidly, and don't mind taking you down with them—and these are your own cells! They have gone over to the dark side. But, believe it or not, cancer is being prevented day in and day out by **you**, by the genetic programs hidden deep within the cell itself (Welsh, 2007). *This* better be going well! And, most of the time, it is.

When cellular growth is improperly regulated, cancer can occur. When a cancer cell makes its debut, there are genetic programs within that are able to detect this abnormal state and rapidly correct the situation. And wouldn't you know, vitamin D regulates the performance of many of these important genetic programs (Spina et al., 2006; Welsh, 2007). Furthermore, there are certain specialized cells (i.e., lymphocytes, aka white blood cells) that move freely about the body and are programmed to notice the "strange goings on" of other cells and target them for destruction (Mariani et al., 1999). It just so happens, vitamin D regulates the performance of these cancer-fighting

~ 34 ~

cells, too! In addition, by **1)** promoting healthy cell division and cellular differentiation (Sutton and MacDonald, 2003), **2)** by limiting the growth of a blood supply (angiogenesis), one capable of supporting the explosive growth of cancer cells (Holick, 2007), **3)** by inhibiting the ability of a cancer cell to successfully metastasize (Holick, 2006a; Spina et al., 2006), and **4)** by regulating the ability of a cell to self-destruct (apoptosis) when things go wrong (Holick, 2004a; Holick 2006a), vitamin D is clearly a cancer fighter, no question! Is this science fiction? **No!** It is "business as usual" when things go wrong, dreadfully wrong, at the cellular level. This regulation of normal cellular performance, and even the beneficial, self-inflected death of a cancer cell (called apoptosis), cell by cell, is all regulated by the hormone we call a vitamin. You did not know this, but all this good depends on vitamin D availability (Lappe et al., 2007; Wagner et al., 2008). When vitamin D is in adequate supply, your risk of many, many cancers (15 different cancers, according to Wagner et al., 2008) goes down significantly. I have some surprising statistics to share:

- "A pooled analysis of studies that assessed serum 25D in relation to breast cancer demonstrated a clear dose-response relationship, with the highest quintile [upper one fifth] of serum 25D associated with a **50% reduction in breast cancer risk**." (Welsh, 2007, emphasis added)

- "It has been suggested that maintenance of a 25(OH)D level greater than 20 ng/ml reduces the risk of colon, prostate, breast, and ovarian cancer by as much as **30–50%**." (Holick, 2006b, emphasis added)

- "Children exposed to the most sunlight had a **40% reduced risk** of developing non-Hodgkin lymphoma." (Holick, 2006b, emphasis added)

- "Tuohimaa et al reported that the risk of prostate cancer was **reduced by 50%** with serum 25(OH)D concentrations of >50 nmol/l [>20 ng/ml]." (Holick, 2004b, emphasis added)

If you are serious about preventing cancer (and who wouldn't be), become very serious about achieving and maintaining a respectable vitamin D level. Not only can vitamin D prevent some cancers that have a strong genetic component (Welsh, 2007), it can also prevent some cancers that are caused by carcinogens supplied to us by our compromised environment (Welsh, 2007). In one study, an enhanced vitamin D status greatly improved the 5-year survival rate of early-stage lung cancer patients (Grimes, 2006). So it is clear, vitamin D sufficiency offers us a significant degree of protection from one of the most dreaded of all diseases, the one we call cancer (although I can certainly think of others that are at least equally dreadful). Cancer takes away so very much if given the chance—actually, it can take away everything! This disease alone should *compel* us to become vitamin D sufficient. Let's move on to the next disease—I've had it with cancer!

Serious about preventing cancer?

Let's hope you are. Since knowledge is power (and motivates you to take action), perhaps you should watch these excellent online videos:

—**Vitamin D Prevents Cancer: Is It True?**
www.youtube.com/watch?v=TQ-qekFoi-o&reature=channel

—**Vitamin D Is Awesome for Cancer**
www.youtube.com/watch?v=foc9gil8OLM&feature=related

—**How Vitamin D Reduces Incidence of Cancer: DINOMIT Model**
www.youtube.com/watch?v=3GM0CnO6-ds&NR=1

Comment: This last video is a little heavy on the science, but you can still learn from it. I believe every physician should watch this one. Links to the above videos, and more, are available on my website.

On a personal note . . .

Recall, I am a recovery room nurse. (Sometimes this job kinda breaks your heart.) Recently (yesterday) I took care of two very sweet young ladies (mid-30s), immediately post op. I was deeply impressed with both and felt that it was indeed an honor to be their nurse. Even though they were *very* brave and had a clear sense of relief that their ordeal would soon be over, I could not help but detect their sadness over what life had handed to them. This is their story:

One lady had been diagnosed with cancer in one breast earlier in the year and subsequently had a mastectomy in order to save her life. On the day I took care of her, she had the other breast removed as a precautionary measure. How sad! How life changing! The other lady I received from surgery this same day had just had both breasts surgically removed due to her genetic markers and a strong family history of breast cancer. She did not have cancer herself, but was advised that this was the prudent thing to do (in order to prevent what seemed to be the inevitable). Talk about a tough decision to make! Was any attention to vitamin D paid at any time on behalf of these ladies in the past? I do not know. Should it have been? I'll let you judge for yourself. But I can tell you that cancer is one nightmare you can live without. Vitamin D sufficiency can, without question and in great measure, prevent the nightmare we call cancer, even breast cancer. Ladies, I would pay close attention to the content of this gray box. Be serious about breast cancer prevention. One out of seven ladies today will have to deal with this disease at some point in their life unless I have something to say about it. At least watch the first two of the three videos listed at the beginning of this gray box and I won't have to track you down and get after you. **Do I look like I'm kidding?**

Iodine and breast cancer

It's not all about vitamin D. Adequate iodine nutrition also reduces the risk of breast cancer. Iodine is intimately involved in breast health and acts to suppress the development of breast cancer. This assertion is supported by the fact that in the Japanese culture there is a much lower incidence of breast cancer than is found in Western cultures, and high levels of dietary iodine intake certainly deserve at least some of the credit. So it should come as no surprise that I believe iodine supplementation should be promoted as a measure to prevent this disease. (The use of iodized salt is simply not enough.) And I am not alone in this opinion. The following paper, written for the layperson, tells the story exceptionally well:

—**Piccone N** 2011 The Silent Epidemic of Iodine Deficiency. www.lef.org/magazine/mag2011/oct2011_The-Silent-Epidemic-of-Iodine-Deficiency_01.htm

Chapter 7
Diabetes

A clearer example of an autoimmune disease that is regulated by the vitamin D hormone is type 1 diabetes mellitus.   ~**DeLuca, 2004**

VDRs are present in pancreatic β-cells and vitamin D is <u>essential</u> for normal insulin secretion.

Increased vitamin D intake during pregnancy significantly reduced β-cell autoimmunity in offspring as directed by islet autoantibodies.
~**Mathieu and Badenhoop, 2005, emphasis added**

Vitamin D supplementation in infancy seems to exert a strong protective effect against the autoimmune disease type I diabetes, and vitamin D levels in early childhood could also have an impact on the risk of MS.   ~**Munger et al., 2006**

*Astonishingly, they found that children who received vitamin D supplementation at the recommended 2,000 IU/d had **reduced the risk of developing diabetes type 1 by 80%**.*   ~**Holick, 2002, emphasis added**

*Recently, Hypponen et al. reported the results of a large birth-cohort study highlighting the importance of vitamin D supplementation for the prevention of diabetes mellitus type I in children. Their data clearly showed that regular vitamin D intake compared with no supplementation during the first year of life was associated with an **88% risk reduction** of type I diabetes mellitus in later life. Even children who received vitamin D irregularly had an **84% lower risk** than those with no supplementation.*
~**Peterlik and Cross, 2005, emphasis added**

Vitamin D deficiency in utero and during the first year of life has also been linked to increased risk of type 1 diabetes. 1,25(OH)$_2$D affects the immune system, and, as pancreatic islet β cell have a VDR, it also *stimulates insulin secretion. Thus, hypovitaminosis D in children may increase their risk not only of type 2 diabetes but also insulin resistance and islet β cell dysfunction.* **~Holick, 2006**

Another study showed that a combined daily intake of 1200 mg of calcium and 800 IU of vitamin D lowered the risk of type 2 diabetes by 33% . . . as compared with a daily intake of less than 600 mg of calcium and less than 400 IU of vitamin D. **~Holick, 2007**

Yes, the risk of diabetes is elevated in those who live a life deficient in vitamin D. Children are at increased risk type 1 diabetes—even type 2 diabetes—should they be deficient. As for the adult, his or her vitamin D status can also be a strong contributing factor in the development of type 2 diabetes, even type 1. It is becoming increasingly clear that the immune system, compromised by a lack of the hormone we call a vitamin, plays a significant role in the development of diabetes, regardless of type. Let's take a look. We'll start first with type 1 diabetes. Alarmingly, in the United States over 15,000 children per year are diagnosed as having this disease!

Regarding the far-reaching effects of vitamin D deficiency, experienced during the earliest phase of life, the following has been written: *"Vitamin D deficiency in pregnancy probably increases the incidence of autoimmune diseases, such as type 1 diabetes, in genetically predisposed individuals."* (Mathieu and Badenhoop, 2005) This has been clearly demonstrated in mice models of type 1 diabetes and certainly applies to humans as well. **In mice, type 1 diabetes can be created, or prevented, <u>100%</u> of the time just by manipulating their vitamin D status, even before birth** (Zella and DeLuca, 2003; Mathieu and Badenhoop, 2005). Regarding humans, the following has been written:

A major clinical lesson that can be drawn at this moment is that avoidance of vitamin D deficiency is essential for β-cell function, and might contribute to protection against type 1 diabetes in later life. (Mathieu and Badenhoop, 2005)

The β cell, mentioned above, is the insulin-producing cell of the pancreas; and during the course of type 1 diabetes its function becomes impaired and the cell itself is destroyed by the individual's own immune system (and a life is forever changed). It certainly appears that vitamin D sufficiency can help prevent this unfortunate turn of events, and for many, many reasons. Vitamin D prevents inappropriate immune responses and helps the immune system ward off attack from bacteria, the two issues that are regarded as fundamental to the development of type 1 diabetes. Now let's turn our attention to type 2 diabetes.

Type 2 diabetes also claims a lot of victims, *"with more than 1 million new cases per year diagnosed in the United States alone.* **Diabetes is the _fifth_ leading cause of death in the United States,** *and it is also a major cause of significant morbidity."* (Pittas et al., 2007, emphasis added) Fifteen million Americans have the disease and approximately five million more could be added to this list but have yet to be diagnosed (Pradhan et al., 2001). Who would *not* want to put a dent in these statistics? Who would *not* want to prevent the growing incidence of this very serious disease? **You can!** It's called vitamin D sufficiency as a way of life.

There are many factors, to be sure, that contribute to the development of diabetes—genetics, diet, weight around the middle— but a low vitamin D status is certainly in there somewhere. It may be surprising to learn that chronic, low-grade inflammation is strongly related to the development of type 2 diabetes, a form of diabetes that is associated with an ongoing, inflammatory-mediated insulin resistance in certain cells throughout the body, and, to some extent, is associated with an increased loss or dysfunction of the insulin-producing β cells themselves (Pittas et al., 2007).

> An accumulating body of evidence suggests that inflammation may play a crucial intermediary role in pathogenesis, thereby linking diabetes with a number of commonly coexisting conditions thought to originate through inflammatory mechanisms. (Pradhan et al., 2001)

Vitamin D, by its ability to favorably influence the immune system, is believed to prevent the development of diabetes in children, young adults, older adults, and mice of all ages—*if* supplies are adequate. There is so much to say regarding the relationship between low vitamin D status and diabetes, but we have to move on—I'm trying to keep things brief (something very hard for me to do). Word of advice: Become vitamin D sufficient as a way of life and you may prevent this disease, delay its onset, or perhaps lessen the severity of its course should you have contracted this serious, oftentimes deadly disease. But should we consider more than vitamin D in the battle against diabetes?

Walking away from diabetes

Yes, you can do this . . . possibly, maybe. There are many approaches to take should one wish to leave this disease in the dust. Exercise is one approach. Diet, of course, is another. Combine the two, and you have a much better chance for success. What is clear is that our modern lifestyle, particularly the lack of adequate energy expenditure in the face of caloric excess, contributes greatly to the incidence and persistence of type 2 diabetes. In keeping with this, both walking and dieting are recommended to prevent, help reverse, or lessen the severity of this disease. I personally have met individuals who were diabetics but are diabetics no longer, some having accomplished this feat by exercise alone, some by diet alone, and some by both diet and exercise. As I recall, two individuals in particular lost between 20 and 25 pounds each, are both off insulin, and are no longer considered diabetic. Would you like to join them? Walking briskly, say 30 to 60 minutes a day, may be all that it takes. This is a great way to change your life, and if you walk between late morning and mid-afternoon, depending on the season (and the amount of clothing you wear), you can easily meet your vitamin D needs for the day, and perhaps for many days to follow. And I'm not just talkin' adults, I'm talkin' kids, too! *"Particularly disturbing is the 10-fold increase in incidences of type 2 diabetes among children between 1982 and 1994."* (Hill et al., 2003) Consider the following:

> Given the many health benefits of physical activity, participation in a regular activity routine is of primary importance and encouraged for individuals with type 1 and type 2 diabetes as well as for those with prediabetes. (American Association of Diabetes Educators, 2012)

The following papers may help get you motivated. Consider reading:

—**Loreto CD, Fanelli C, Lucidi P, Murdolo G, De Cicco A, Parlanti N, Ranchelli A, et al** 2005 Make Your Diabetic Patients Walk. Diabetes Care 28(6):1295–1302

—**Hill JO** 2005 Walking and Type 2 Diabetes. Diabetes Care 28(6):1524–1525

—**Albright A** 2005 Moving Ahead with Physical Activity. Diabetes Spectrum 18(2):86–87

As important as exercise (and diet) is to the management of diabetes, there may be something of equal importance to consider.

Iron and diabetes

> Mounting evidence suggests that increased body iron stores are involved in the pathogenesis of insulin-resistant disorders such as the metabolic syndrome and type 2 diabetes in the general population. (Martíez-Garcia et al., 2009)

There is a surprising (and largely ignored) relationship between iron and diabetes. And you live in a world that just can't wait to give you all the iron that you don't need. Please, pay close attention. Due to iron fortification of refined and prepared foods, red meat in abundance, iron supplements—even water supplies that contain relatively high levels of iron—our society is experiencing the serious problem of iron excess. As a result, the cells of the pancreas are challenged, damaged, and our risk of diabetes has become elevated.

Iron is truly a "double-edged sword." We need it so badly—and you certainly do not want to become or remain anemic from iron deficiency—but, when in excess of individual need and in context with any compromise in the ability to cope with iron accumulation at the tissue and cell level, we get into trouble. Diabetes is trouble—both type 1 and type 2. Strong evidence for a role of iron in the pathogenesis and perpetuation of diabetes can be found in the following papers. The first one is the most compelling, a must read (unless you don't want to).

—**Fernández-Real JM, López-Bernejo A, Richart W** 2002 Cross-Talk Between Iron and Diabetes. Diabetes 51:2348–2354

—**Jiang R, Manson JE, Meigs JB, Ma J, Rifai N, Hu FB** 2004 Body Iron Stores in Relation to Risk of Type 2 Diabetes in Apparently Healthy Women. JAMA; February 11; 291(6):711–717

—**Swaminathan S, Fonseca S, Alam MG, Shah SV** 2007 The Role of Iron in Diabetes and Its Complications. Diabetes Care; July; 30(7):1926–1933

—**Ashraf AP, Eason NB, Kabagamble EK, Haritha EK, Meleth S, McCormick KL** 2010 Dietary Iron Intake in the First 4 Months of Infancy and the Development of Type 1 Diabetes: A Pilot Study. Diabetology & Metabolic Syndrome 2(58):1–7

The papers listed above (and there are many more I could list) tell a story, an important but somewhat neglected story. I want you, dear diabetic patient, to print out these papers, read them, hand them to your physician, and together come up with a plan that will address the issue of iron excess and diabetes. When diet and exercise is not enough, perhaps taking measures that reduce iron stores will do the trick.

On a personal note: I do not have diabetes. I do not plan to have diabetes. (But if I did have diabetes, I would fight it tooth and nail.) So, in order to reduce my risk, I am intentionally limiting my dietary iron intake. But I do something else that is certain to help. I regularly donate blood in order to reduce my tissue iron stores, and thereby reduce my risk of diabetes and other diseases, like Parkinson's disease, like Alzheimer's disease, like cancer, and like cardiovascular disease. Yes, a reduction in tissue iron stores, via blood donation and/or a substantial limitation of dietary iron, can help reduce one's risk of several debilitating age-related diseases. With respect to type 2 diabetes, people can reduce their insulin need and improve their diabetic state simply by donating blood to those in need (Fernández-Real, et al., 2002). I would pay attention to this! Diabetes may seem okay and easy to manage at first, but I see trouble ahead. *Never* let diabetes become acceptable! Try to find a way out. Addressing the iron/diabetes issue might just give you an edge. (But don't forget about vitamin D.) Consider the following:

> High iron stores . . . are associated with an increased risk of type 2 diabetes in healthy women independent of known diabetes risk factors. (Jiang et al., 2004)

> In 1969, Williams et al. showed that diabetic patients treated with phlebotomy [think blood donation] required less insulin than similar patients during the phlebotomy period. In 1972 Dymock et al. reported a significant reduction in total daily insulin dosage following phlebotomy.

> Simple and inexpensive therapies, such as bloodletting and iron chelators, are emerging as alternative and effective treatments for insulin resistance. (Fernández-Real, et al., 2002)

> Blood donation is simultaneously associated with increased insulin sensitivity and decreased iron stores. Stored iron seems to impact negatively on insulin action even in healthy people, and not just in classic pathological conditions associated with iron overload. (Fernández-Real, et al., 2005)

Diabetes and gastric bypass

Believe it or not, diabetes type 2 can be cured by surgery in those who also are obese. In a majority of cases, the diabetic state is gone in a matter of days! Occasionally, gastric bypass is performed, not necessarily for the weight loss, but for the termination of diabetes. There are lessons to be learned here. Generally, obesity equals insulin resistance. And, generally, weight loss equals improved insulin sensitivity. Even those who are not considered obese but have pounds to spare can benefit from weight loss, and benefit in many, many ways.

Chapter 8
Autoimmune disease

Autoimmune diseases are the <u>third leading cause of morbidity and mortality in the industrialized world</u>, surpassed only by cancer and heart disease. **~Arnson et al., 2007, emphasis added**

The active form of vitamin D is a potent regulator of the immune system. **~VanAmerongen et al., 2004**

The effects of $1\alpha,25(OH)_2D_3$ on the immune system are multiple, but all lead to the generation of tolerance and anergy [lack of response] rather than immune activation. **~Mathieu and Badenhoop, 2005**

Among whites, there was a <u>41% decrease in MS risk for every 50 nmol/L increase in 25-hydroxyvitamin D</u>. **~Munger et al., 2006, emphasis added**

Mounting evidence indicates a high prevalence of vitamin D deficiency in the general population, and this deficiency has been linked to an increased incidence of autoimmune diseases, as well as bone diseases and cancer. Epidemiological analysis reveals strong ecological and case-controlled evidence that the vitamin D system reduces the risk of several autoimmune diseases, including multiple sclerosis (MS), type 1 diabetes, inflammatory bowel disease (IBD), RA [rheumatoid arthritis], osteoarthritis, and SLE [lupus]. **~Adorini and Penna, 2008**

Every experimental model of autoimmunity tested (experimental MS, inflammatory bowel disease, type 1 diabetes, arthritis, lupus, etc.) show sensitivity to vitamin D status and/or suppression of symptoms. **~Cantorna, 2008**

Autoimmunity occurs when the immune system becomes misdirected and recognizes a part of *you* as "foreign," and inflicts great damage on specific target tissues and cells, the ones that seem particularly vulnerable to attack or the ones that simply get in the way. It just so happens that you are at greater risk for an autoimmune disease should you be deficient in vitamin D. The genetics and dynamics in play here are so incredibly complex, but sunshine exposure and taking vitamin D supplements are not. Multiple sclerosis (MS) is but one of many autoimmune diseases associated with vitamin D deficiency. I don't like it at all. So we'll start with this disease in our brief discussion of autoimmunity.

Multiple sclerosis

The prevalence of MS is nearly zero close to the equator and is markedly increased in regions of more northern latitudes. **~Zittermann, 2003**

Early sun avoidance seems to precede the diagnosis of multiple sclerosis (MS). This protective effect is independent of genetic susceptibility to MS. **~Islam et al., 2007, emphasis added**

Early life sunlight exposure and dietary vitamin D supplementation diminish the risk of MS. **~Chaudhuri, 2005**

Living above the 35° latitude [above Los Angeles or Atlanta, for example] for the first 10 years of life imprints on a child for the rest of his or her life a **100% increased risk** *[double the risk] of developing multiple sclerosis no matter where they live thereafter.* **~Holick 2006, emphasis added**

Another study checked the vitamin D intake in more than 187,000 women from two separate cohorts (study groups) . . . and found a 40% reduction in the risk of multiple sclerosis among women who used supplemental vitamin D. **~Arnson et al., 2007**

The prevalence of MS is highest where environmental supplies of vitamin D are lowest. It is well recognized that the active hormone form of

vitamin D . . . is a natural immunoregulator with anti-inflammatory action.
~VanAmerongen et al., 2004

Mice that were pretreated with 1,25(OHO)$_2$D-3 before they were injected with myelin to induce a multiple-sclerosis like disease were immune from it. ~Holick, 2005

Multiple sclerosis (MS) results from what appears to be a progressive autoimmune attack on the insulation that covers the nerves within the central nervous system. The attack damages and degrades the myelin sheath, and results in a variety of physical disabilities, disabilities generally related to the inability of the affected nerves to conduct nerve impulses. Under the circumstances, the messages the brain sends forth just cannot get through. The cause of this disease is yet to be determined, but genetics, perhaps an opportunistic pathogen, and the environment seem to all come together and alter a life forever. But we do know this: MS is so closely related to a lack of sunlight exposure that it is crazy! We'd better shine a little (sun)light on the disease we call MS.

It seems that all you need is a genetic predisposition and, in the context of vitamin D insufficiency, your risk of coming down with one very nasty disease becomes significantly elevated. Yet this disease is in the *"very preventable"* range! (Hayes et al., 1997; Hayes et al., 2003) In fact, the genetic predisposition may take a back seat to hypovitaminosis D when it comes to developing MS (Hayes et al., 1997; Orton et al., 2008). Case in point: If you have a twin, one with identical genetics, and become separated at birth (story to appear on *60 Minutes*), with *you* staying in a sunny region to receive *"2 to 3 hours of youthful sun exposure on average per week"* and your twin going up north (to be an indoor person), your twin has a **60% greater risk** of contracting MS than you do (Islam et al., 2007). This is a fairly significant finding! Another example: If, on the other hand, you are an unfortunate mouse with vitamin D deficiency, and you have a twin mousie (yes, this is a word), one that maintains a vitamin D level that is sufficient—and both you and your twin are given experimental MS—you have a **100%** chance of coming down with MS. Your twin, however, will have a **100%** chance of _not_ developing MS and going on to have a lot more fun in life than you (Hayes et al., 1997; Hayes, 2000; Holick, 2005). *You* are one *very* unlucky mouse!

In view of the studies revealing a strong association between hypovitaminosis D and the incidence of MS, one cannot help but wonder if we as a society are just letting this disease happen. Where are the public service announcements and ad campaigns warning us of the increased risk of MS should one continue to live a life deficient in vitamin D? Such announcements and warnings are nowhere to be found. Yet this is a disease that affects 2.5 million people worldwide and claims thousands of new American victims each year! No, I'm not seeing a sense of urgency in our society directed at the prevention of one very debilitating disease. And as for its treatment, I certainly hope that the physician who is caring for the MS patient has read the following: *"Once MS is apparent, low 25(OH)D levels may aggravate its severity."* (VanAmerongen et al., 2004) In light of what we know about the relationship between vitamin D and MS—the prevention and treatment—much attention is now given to this issue. I hope it's enough.

In one study, 5,000 IU of vitamin D per day, along with calcium and magnesium supplementation, reduced exacerbations in MS patients by **59%** compared with previous year(s) (VanAmerongen et al., 2004). I'm liking the sound of this!

In conclusion: If you have MS (or just want to prevent one nasty disease), take notice of vitamin D. Find out all you can! And take the steps necessary to become vitamin D sufficient, under physician guidance and approval of course. With respect to MS, it is important to realize that vitamin D regulates several genetic events associated with both myelination and remyelination after insult and injury (Chaudhuri, 2005; Spach et al., 2004; Potera, 2009). And, yes, remyelination of damaged neurons does occur in MS, at least on a limited basis (Boccaccio and Steinman, 1996; Chaudhuri, 2005; Franco et al., 2008;

McTigue and Tripathi, 2008). If you have MS, it is doubtful that you will benefit at all from hypovitaminosis D.

Rheumatoid arthritis (RA)

RA is an immune-mediated disease characterized by articular inflammation and subsequent tissue damage, which can lead to severe disability and subsequent tissue damage. **~Adorina and Penna, 2008**

An inflammatory reaction is thought to underlie the joint pathology seen in chronic arthritis, namely, thickening of the synovial lining with increased vascularization and ultimately, irreversible damage to cartilage and bone. **~Cantorna et al., 1998**

An increase in vitamin D has been associated with decreased risk of developing rheumatoid arthritis. **~Holick, 2004**

Rheumatoid arthritis was another example of an inflammatory arthritis that can be largely prevented by the administration of the vitamin D compounds. **~Durmus et al., 2012**

Well, let's look at what we do with this disease, a disease that is caused by an immune system attack on various joints of the body, causing pain, stiffness, and loss of mobility. The joints are not the only target of this disease, RA can also effect many other parts of the body, producing a wide variety of symptoms ranging from unpleasant to devastating. It can actually kill (Kelly and Hamilton, 2006). We seldom take measures to prevent this disease, perhaps uncertain what steps we should take. And, when the disease strikes, we use drugs that help (but can also harm)—out of necessity! That's just about it. One class of drugs called NSAIDs (e.g., Aleve, Motrin, Ibuprofen, Aspirin), commonly used to treat the pain and inflammation of rheumatoid arthritis as well as other inflammatory conditions permanently kills 7,000 to 10,000 Americans each year! (Lanza et al., 2009) (Death, of course, should be thought of as harmful.) Yet this class of drugs, and others, <u>are needed</u>, and the risks are accepted when the immediate and long-term goal is to put the brakes on the inflammatory process and prevent further damage. Less—perhaps much less—of this rheumatoid arthritis business would be occurring if we paid more attention in our society to vitamin D. Studies have shown that vitamin D adequacy can go a long way in preventing this disease. And, even if you have contracted this disease, vitamin D still may help! *"Recently, greater intake of vitamin D was associated with a lower risk of RA, as well as a significant clinical improvement was correlated with the immunomodulating potential in vitamin D-treated RA patients."* (Cutolo et al., 2007) It would be very hard for me not to suggest that the rheumatoid arthritis patient have a vitamin D level drawn to see if vitamin D deficiency is present, and to have it corrected as indicated . . . particularly after reading the following:

> In patients with RA measuring vitamin D levels seems particularly pertinent as deficiency is highly prevalent in this group. Vitamin D may also have a role in modulating RA disease activity and is already known to be important in osteoporosis and falls, which are common in RA. (Leventis and Patel, 2008)

Lupus (SLE)

> *Vitamin D deficiency is a risk factor for SLE, and reduced serum levels of $1,25(OH)_2D_3$ in patients with SLE might contribute to the β-cell hyperactivity observed in this disease.* **~Adorini and Penna, 2008**

> *There may be a higher vitamin D requirement for patients at risk for developing autoimmune disease and for those that already have an autoimmune disease such as systemic lupus erythematosus.* **~Cutolo et al., 2007**

Surprisingly, lupus, like MS, seems to be in the preventable range, preventable by a life enriched by vitamin D. And, like MS, its course may be modified by maintaining a sufficient level of vitamin D in the affected individual (Adorini and Penna, 2008). I doubt if 600 IU/d is going to cut it here—just not enough! (But it could, per individual circumstances and physiologic need.)

Lupus, like both MS and rheumatoid arthritis, is considered to be the result of autoimmunity. Like these and other diseases falling into this category, lupus can be quite challenging to manage. It is often difficult to diagnose, as it presents with a wide variety of symptoms leading to destruction and disrupted function in a variety of tissues, organs, and systems. If not recognized early or treated appropriately, this disease can lead to serious heart and kidney ailments. And with respect to vitamin D and the lupus patient, the issues are quite complex.

For example, one of the drugs used to treat lupus, HCQ (hydroxychloroquine, aka Plaquenil), may elevate an individual's 25(OH)D$_3$ level making it appear that all is well, but this drug inhibits the enzyme that converts 25(OH)D$_3$ into the active form of vitamin D, the 1,25 form that helps regulate the immune system (Ruiz-Irastorza et al., 2008). Thus, hydroxychloroquine (Plaquenil) creates a subtle form of vitamin D deficiency. In addition, the individual with lupus is also at risk, perhaps even greater risk, of other diseases that are clearly influenced by vitamin D. So vitamin D adequacy for the one with this disease just makes sense. The hope is, of course, with vitamin D replacement the individual will have a kinder and gentler lupus to deal with and no other problems will emerge. But, wouldn't you know, there are other vitamin D-related problems the lupus patient may experience.

The lupus patient may exhibit an intolerance to sunlight (Ruiz-Irastorza et al., 2008). Sunlight avoidance therefore becomes a necessity, but unfortunately this course of action, while appropriate, deprives the individual of the primary source of vitamin D. And, of course, the individual's vitamin D status is at risk of further compromise. The vitamin D status of the lupus patient should probably be closely followed and not be considered to be of only casual concern.

Treatment of vitamin D deficiency is particularly important in patients with SLE due to other concomitant insults on their bones and in view of the possible immunomodulatory effects of vitamin D. Therefore it is important to consider the possibility of vitamin D deficiency. (Barnes and Bucknall, 2004)

Let's end this chapter something like this:

There are a variety of autoimmune diseases from which to choose. I would not choose any one of them. Some are relatively easy to manage and may not even be noticeable at first. On the other hand, some are quite severe, and a life is never ever the same. Vitamin D sufficiency has been shown to prevent autoimmunity, in good measure, if supplies are adequately maintained. Are you listening? Vitamin D sufficiency allows nice things to happen.

The active form of vitamin D produces and maintains self immunologic tolerance, some studies show that 1,25(OH)2D inhibits induction of disease in autoimmune encephalomyelitis, thyroiditis, type-1 diabetes mellitus, inflammatory bowel disease (IBD), systemic lupus erythematosus, and collagen-induced arthritis and Lyme arthritis. (Ginanjar et al., 2007)

The following sums things up quite nicely:

The common denominator that rises from these studies is that vitamin D affects the immune system at many levels and by a number of mechanisms. It takes part in the genetic regulation of cytokine production, VDR expression and affects important biological processes by which these cells interact. On the whole, vitamin D confers an immunosuppressive effect. Vitamin D has been shown to provide clinically beneficial effects in animal models, and initial observations indicate that vitamin D supplementation may be preventive in multiple sclerosis and diabetes mellitus. These preliminary results are encouraging and further clinical trials are needed to evaluate the potential role of vitamin D in clinical practice. (Arnson et al., 2007)

A brief word about sarcoidoisis

This disease is a variant of lupus and may lead, not only to sunlight sensitivity and to the overproduction of the active form of vitamin D, but also may lead to serious reactions to supplemental vitamin D. Death, one might say, is a serious reaction. Word of advice: If you have sarcoidosis, get *exceptional* medical attention to help you manage this disease. *Exceptional medical attention* would certainly include a careful evaluation of the issues surrounding vitamin D in you, as an individual.

One more thing to mention about sarcoidosis before we move on, —and this is important! In sarcoidosis, high blood levels of calcium (hypercalcemia) can occur in response to sunlight exposure or in response to vitamin D ingestion. This is a serious matter and can lead to severe complications. Apparently, in this disease, an inappropriate blood level of the "active" vitamin D hormone is produced by the cells involved in the disease process. This does not always happen, but it can! And I quote:

> Depending on the population studied about 2–63% of sarcoidosis patients show hypercalcemia. The major difference in the prevalence of hypercalcemia may be due to the undulating course of subacute sarcoidosis, so hypercalcemia may be missed when serum calcium is not frequently measured. Hypercalciuria [high calcium in the urine] appears to be twice as prevalent than hypercalcemia and should be looked for in every sarcoidosis patient. Hypercalcemia in sarcoidosis is due to the uncontrolled synthesis of 1,25-dihydroxyvitamin D3 by macrophages [a type of immune cell]. 1,25-dihydroxyvitamin D3 leads to an increased absorption of calcium in the intestine and to an increased resorption of calcium in the bone. . . . It is thought that 1,25-dihydroxyvitamin D3 counter regulates uncontrolled granuloma formation. Treatment of hypercalcemia depends on the serum level of hypercalcemia and its persistence. Generally sarcoidotic patients should avoid sun exposure to reduce vitamin D3 synthesis, to omit fish oils that are rich in vitamin D and to produce more than two liters of urine a day by adapting fluid intake. (Ackerman, 2007)

I showcase sarcodoisis here in order to get this point across: If you have a serious disease, or distressing symptoms that have yet to be explained, you *will* need medical guidance with respect to vitamin D supplementation. No question. If you go out on your own here, I see trouble ahead (but then, I always see trouble ahead). Even though vitamin D may help prevent a particular disease like lupus, once the disease process is in full swing, vitamin D may or may not help; in fact it might even make things worse. Sarcodosis teaches us this very important lesson. I'm all for vitamin D, but I'm all for exercising caution when it comes to vitamin D, too, depending, of course, on the circumstances.

Chapter 9
Inflammatory bowel disease

Vitamin D deficiency has been linked to several different diseases, including the immune-system diseases ulcerative colitis and Crohn's disease. **~Cantorna et al., 2004**

Autoimmune diseases are diseases where the immune system's ability to discriminate between self- and non-self tissue fails. People with diseases like multiple sclerosis (MS), arthritis, and inflammatory bowel disease (IBD) have T cells that target self and drive the immune system to induce inflammation in the peripheral tissues. **~Cutolo et al., 2007**

Living at higher latitudes increases the risk of type 1 diabetes, multiple sclerosis, and Crohn's disease. **~Holick, 2007**

Patients with a defect in the mucosa may experience a higher risk of microbial infection, for example, which may trigger the onset of IBD in patients that are predisposed. Our study showed that vitamin D is able to strengthen the mucosal barrier by upregulating some of the key tight junction proteins. **In a vitamin D-deficient state, mucosal barriers are more susceptible to injury that leads to infection and IBD.** **~Liu, 2008, emphasis added**

Y ou may be wondering why inflammatory bowel disease (IBD) was not included in the previous chapter, the chapter on autoimmune disease. There *is* a good reason. Although generally regarded as autoimmune, IBD seems to be in a class all by itself. And at least one of the diseases that fall under this heading, Crohn's disease (CD), is not an autoimmune disease at all! It is something else. Ulcerative colitis (UC), however, is still considered to be autoimmune, but that could change at any moment. Now back to Crohn's. Rather than being an autoimmune disease, Crohn's is, in all likelihood, an immunodeficiency disease (Kelsall, 2008; Yamamoto-Furusho and Korzenik, 2006). In case you were wondering, I do know this subject well. I wrote a book on Crohn's disease. I'll tell you more, later. But now let's take a look at the intimate relationship between vitamin D and IBD. We'll start with Crohn's. And I'll try to keep this under 500 pages.

Crohn's disease (CD)

Compromise or disruption of the intestinal barrier function causes deleterious effects and results in exposure of the host to luminal antigens and bacteria, leading to inflammation.

These observations suggest that VDR plays a critical role in mucosal barrier homeostasis by preserving the integrity of junctions complexes and healing capacity of the colonic epithelium. **~Kong et al., 2008**

In summary, mucosal innate immunodeficiency characterized by impaired dysfunction of neutrophils, monocytes and dendritic cells [all key cells of the immune system] as well as intestinal epithelium play a key role in the development of CD. **~Yamamoto-Furusho and Korzenik, 2006**

As mentioned, Crohn's disease is not an autoimmune disease, as was once thought. It may be more accurately characterized as an immunodeficiency disease. This is important! The body is not attacking itself, although this does seem to be the case; rather, the immune system, or a part thereof, is struggling to perform. During the course of this disease, the tissues of the bowel are adversely affected by ongoing inflammation. Pain, bleeding, and diarrhea come and go, people get better, and then they get unbetter, and eventually most— approximately 80%—will need some form of intestinal surgery at least once in their lifetime. Unfortunately, many requiring surgical intervention will walk out of the hospital with a bag attached to collect stool, a situation that will last the remainder of their lives. You really don't want this disease. And if you have it you can't <u>wait</u> for it to go away. It is typically treated with powerful drugs, drugs that oftentimes stop the madness but sometimes fail to perform, and can lead to severe complications including the severe complication of death. Even Medicine is disappointed with what it has to offer the individual with this disease. Too bad vitamin D deficiency may have contributed to the individual's susceptibility. People are clearly more at risk of contracting Crohn's when they are low in vitamin D.

The fundamental problem recently identified in Crohn's is an impaired ability to clear (destroy) pathogens, pathogens that somehow penetrate the surface lining (epithelium) of the bowel and take up residence within the macrophage, a key immune cell that lives and moves about beneath this epithelial barrier. Its job is to find, devour, then kill the pathogen that has dared enter this tissue region. The devouring goes well, but the killing does not. Surprisingly, if the pathogen can obtain enough iron from the host cell, it can continue to exist, replicate, and stir up all kinds of trouble (Nairz et al., 2010). In Crohn's, the inflammatory response continues and must be suppressed. Accordingly, medications are prescribed to accomplish this feat. But perhaps it would be wise to prevent the offender from obtaining or utilizing iron. This can be done. Incidentally, iron withholding is the central theme of my book on Crohn's. The book also features the alternative and complementary approaches appropriate for the management of this disease.

Sorry! I didn't mean to put a plug in for my book. (Okay, I did—but it is a very good book, and my cat is on the verge of starvation . . . please help.) And, yes, the book has one "killer" of a chapter on vitamin D. Actually, vitamin D plays a vital role in killing the pathogen that thinks it is safely hidden from danger (Nerich et al., 2011; Liu et at., 2008). For this reason, and for many other reasons, Crohn's disease is in the very preventable range. But vitamin D will need to be in adequate supply or you can forget it. Pay attention to the following:

$1,25(OH)_2D_3$ has been shown to act as a potent stimulator of the antibiotic protein cathelicidin (LL37) and thus <u>actively promotes bacterial killing</u> by both macrophages and epithelial cells. (Liu et al., 2008, emphasis added)

There is a wealth of information on the relationship between vitamin D and Crohn's disease. And there are many good reasons to pay close attention. Besides the enhanced killing ability of the immune system afforded by vitamin D sufficiency, vitamin D helps maintain the overall health of the intestinal epithelial surface cell (Kong et al., 2008), a cell that stands between you and trillions of bacteria that would like nothing more than to enter and advance to distant places. But the intestinal epithelial cell is not your ordinary epithelial or surface cell. Believe it or not, **the intestinal epithelial cell is an immune cell!** (Neish, 2002; Mayer, 2000) It can engulf the pathogen, kill it within, or pass it along intact to be killed by any number of other immune cells that live and work nearby, immune cells that live for the kill (Schoultz et al., 2011). The general health of the intestinal epithelial cell, including its ability to defend and to destroy, is dependent on an adequate supply of vitamin D (Sun, 2010). You are clearly more at risk for Crohn's if you are vitamin D deficient. Clearly! But, for ulcerative colitis, things are not so clear.

Ulcerative colitis (UC)

Vitamin D deficiency is common among patients with active UC, particularly those requiring corticosteroids. **~Blanck and Aberra, 2013**

Sunlight and vitamin D might protect against CD by downregulating the T helper (Th) 1-driven immune responses. Consistently, a north-south gradient [presuming north gets less sunlight/vitamin D than south] is <u>not observed</u> for ulcerative colitis, the other major form of inflammatory bowel disease which is considered as a Th2-dominated condition.
~Peyrin-Biroulet et al., 2009, emphasis added

Unlike Crohn's disease, ulcerative colitis is still considered to be an autoimmune disease. The symptoms are often identical to Crohn's. And, as opposed to Crohn's where the battle between pathogen and host is occurring below the intestinal epithelial cell, in ulcerative colitis (UC) the battle is occurring on the surface of the intestinal epithelial cell, typically beginning in the rectum and extending upward to involve the colon.

Normally, luminal bacteria in the gut are withheld from contact with the epithelium by an adherent mucus layer, but in UC the bacteria reside on the luminal surface where they probably induce and maintain the inflammatory process. (Schneider et al., 2010)

Typically, bacteria should <u>not</u> be in contact with the surface of the bowel to any great extent. And, when this does occur and persist, I see trouble ahead . . . as usual. The surface of the bowel is normally protected from contact by a relatively thick layer of mucus, so thick, in fact, that it would take over 2,000 bacteria placed end to end to transverse the intestinal mucous layer (McGuckin et al., 2009; Johansson et al., 2010). Unfortunately, in ulcerative colitis the mucous layer is insufficient to keep bacteria from living and from replicating on the surface lining of the colon, and all hell breaks loose. The fighting (inflammatory response) is intense. And someone could get caught in the crossfire. Somehow, low vitamin D, or altered signaling at the level of the VDR, is important to the pathogenesis of ulcerative colitis (Wang et al., 2010), but, apparently, not all the details have been worked out. This may be the reason why so little information is available on hypovitaminosis D and the risk of contracting ulcerative colitis.

However, a low vitamin D status may impact the life of the one who has this disease, and do so in many, many ways. But don't count on vitamin D to turn things around in a big way once ulcerative colitis has arrived, although it may improve the situation or solve another problem or two (Wang et al., 2010).

One reason that vitamin D supplementation (except in small amounts) may not help the patient with ulcerative colitis is the fact that vitamin D typically intensifies the type of inflammatory response pattern that occurs in ulcerative colitis (Nerich et al., 2011). Accordingly, large amounts of vitamin D may make the disease process in ulcerative colitis more intense. Beware!

And keep this in mind . . .

*Reported side effects of vitamin D include nausea, vomiting, headache, metallic taste, vascular or nephrocalcinosis, and pancreatitis. Reported contraindications to vitamin D include hypercalcemia in sarcoidosis; metastatic bone disease; other granulomatous diseases such as tuberculosis and **Crohn's disease (active phase)** that have a disordered vitamin D metabolism in activated macrophages; and Williams syndrome (infantile hypercalcemia).*   ~**Schwalfenberg, 2007, emphasis added**

I have this concern, a concern shared by many others: During the active phase of Crohn's disease (and possibly ulcerative colitis), vitamin D administration <u>may</u> create another problem you simply do not need. It seems the VDR becomes most active in areas of inflammation and will generate an excess of the active form of vitamin D in the region, the 1,25 form.   This, in turn, will create a "spillover" effect and will introduce an excessive amount of the active vitamin D hormone into the bloodstream (Abreu et al., 2004). This can then lead to any number of adverse effects, and/or the silent loss of bone density (Abreu et al., 2004; Carroll and Schade, 2003).   So be careful with vitamin D supplementation, especially high-dose supplementation in the setting of "active" intestinal inflammation. Wait, as advised by your physician, until the dust settles before attempting to aggressively correct an identified or presumed vitamin D deficiency. This advice applies particularly to Crohn's disease during its active phase, but I am aware of problems that can occur with high-dose vitamin D in the setting of ulcerative colitis. And sometimes ulcerative colitis is misdiagnosed and could actually be Crohn's instead. Therefore, I believe caution should be exercised when it comes to vitamin D supplementation, particularly high-dose supplementation for the patient with "active" ulcerative colitis.

You may want to share this information with someone you know, should they be so unfortunate as to have Crohn's disease or ulcerative colitis. Hey, why not buy them a book?

More to Consider in the Battle against Crohn's

That's the name of my Crohn's book—4 years in the making, nearly 500 pages long, citing over 500 references . . . and quite a story. Crohn's disease is not what you think. **Crohn's disease is war!** This book explains, in layman's terms, exactly what this disease is and how to treat it more effectively. It features the most promising alternative and complementary approaches available in the management of this disease. It also contains information useful to the individual who suffers from ulcerative colitis. There are surprises in store! This really is a unique, one-of-a-kind book on Crohn's. It only exists because of the careful observations that I have made, the unique experiences that have come my way, and a lot of hard work and dedication. And you know me! I like to share. The book will soon be available by special order from my website, as an eBook, or perhaps at your local book store. It will also be for sale on Amazon.com (when I get around to it). For information on the release date and to purchase *More to Consider in the Battle Against Crohn's*, go to:

—**www.impactofvitamind.com**

Chapter 10
Parkinson's disease

Confirmatively, a significant higher prevalence of hypovitaminosis D was observed in patients with Parkinson's disease, when compared to both healthy controls and patients with Alzheimer's disease. **~Fernandes de Abreu et al., 2009**

Vitamin D regulates multiple cellular processes known to be abnormal in Parkinson's disease, including cellular differentiation, proliferation and apoptosis. Additionally, vitamin D receptor and activating enzyme are enriched in hippocampal and substantia nigra cells in the brain, problematic in Parkinson's patients. **~Chorley, 2008**

We are just beginning to notice a close relationship between hypovitaminosis D and Parkinson's disease. Who would have thought, just a few years ago, that research would point us in this direction? I will share with you all I know on the subject. And I'll start with me.

I actually live in fear of any disease named after a person. Parkinson's disease—no exception. Of course, I am basically afraid of any disease regardless of the name, especially those that are no fun at all. Parkinson's disease is no fun at all.

You have probably seen it in action—a little intentional tremor here and a little head bobbing there—and you may think that Parkinson's disease is no big deal. But you would be dead wrong. This thing can *totally* destroy a life! Parkinson's disease generally starts out as mild and annoying. It is generally progressive. Over time, it can wind up producing severe, uncontrollable shaking, particularly of the hands, preventing the individual from eating, drinking, and just about any activity you can think of except mixing paint. And it can lead to dementia, leaving behind a shattered life. Enter vitamin D. Vitamin D sufficiency may help prevent this disease from occurring. Or it may not, but I wouldn't take the chance.

Parkinson's patients are typically found to be low in vitamin D (Evatt et al., 2008)—but, hey, who isn't? So there must be other factors in play that set the stage, like a bacterial or viral insult (Nelson and Paulson, 2002; Whitton, 2007). Iron accumulation and dysregulation are always a factor in the pathogenesis of neurodegenerative diseases such as Parkinson's and Alzheimer's (Sadrzadth and Saffari, 2004). There are certain to be other triggers and other factors involved. And genetics, along with the aging process, must certainly be playing a defining role. One thing the researchers have discovered is that genes *"strongly linked"* to Parkinson's disease are responsive to vitamin D (Fernandes de Abreu et al., 2009). But, then, researchers are always coming up with interesting stuff to tell us. One important discovery: The area of the brain that is affected in Parkinson's disease has <u>the most VDR activity of any other region of the brain</u>! (Fernandes de Abreu et al., 2009) This, of course, would be a very important finding.

When an area of the body has a high number of VDRs, it has a greater need for vitamin D—it's that simple! The VDR, together with vitamin D (in adequate supply), regulates genes, genes that act to maintain normal function, promote tissue repair, and protect against insult, including the insult of inflammation or the insult of an invading pathogen. However, in Parkinson's disease, the insult may actually come from within—no invader needed. It may come from an unfortunate dysregulation of localized brain chemistry (Whitton, 2007). Let me explain.

One event that is regulated by vitamin D involves dealing decisively with the creation and release of nitric oxide by certain brain cells. When the regulation of nitric oxide is impaired, things get a little out of hand—okay, a lot out of hand! Accordingly, excess nitric oxide is produced or a normal production level is not held in check, and damage occurs to both the neuron and the cells that maintain the insulating myelin sheath that protects the neuron (Garcion et al., 2002; Whitton, 2007). Trust me on this one: *This* you do not want! Like MS, the demyelination of neurons occurs in Parkinson's disease (Nelson and Paulson, 2002). Following demyelination, localized scarring takes place and you are left with one very serious problem, one that will dominate your life forever! Your chance of this unfortunate outcome seems to be far greater if the regulatory hormone called vitamin D is in short supply. But even if vitamin D supplies have been adequate, something— perhaps many things yet unidentified—may prevent the local conversion of vitamin D into its most active form, creating a certain degree of "regional" vitamin D deficiency as a result. There are so many unanswered questions here, but it certainly appears that simple vitamin D deficiency, over time, is a contributing factor to the pathogenesis of Parkinson's disease.

So what should we do with this information? Just add it to the list of excellent reasons to become vitamin D sufficient and to remain vitamin D sufficient . . . for life!

Should a bacterium or virus be identified as the cause of Parkinson's, an efficient and effective immune system—supported by adequate vitamin D availability—may be all that it takes to prevent this disease from establishing itself in the first place. On the other hand, once you have the disease, you're probably not going to cure this one with vitamin D!—before the disease becomes evident, too much damage has already been done. However, improvements *may* be made and further damage *may* be prevented should more attention be paid to vitamin D (Newmark and Newmark, 2007). Other diseases, too, will need to be prevented in the individual suffering from Parkinson's. So, while the scientists are busy discovering new things and sorting everything out, why don't we just play it smart and achieve and maintain a respectable vitamin D level, and perhaps prevent this disease from taking hold in the first place? And, should one be so unfortunate as to have the disease, why not see if symptoms abate with adequate vitamin D supplementation?

During my review of the subject, I was able to locate one case report speaking of a significant improvement in the symptoms of Parkinson's disease following supplementation with vitamin D along with supplemental calcium. A summary reads as follows:

> After the addition of 25-(OH) Vit D (4,000 IU daily) and calcium supplements (1 g daily) to the ongoing conventional anti-parkinsonian therapy, serum and urinary calcium and phosphorus values progressively normalized as well as serum 25-(OH) Vit D and 1,25-(OH)$_2$ Vit D values. The Parkinsonism improved significantly during the following year with decreased rigidity and akinesis [difficulty in initiating voluntary movement], and the anti-parkinsonian drugs could be restricted to levodopa 375 mg daily. At 1-year follow-up, neurological examination revealed only moderate rigidity without tremor. (Newmark and Newmark, 2007, emphasis added)

A pacemaker for Parkinson's? Yes, a pacemaker for Parkinson's.

I've seen this thing in action. Works great! I take care of these patients immediately after surgery from time to time. During surgery, an electrical lead is placed into the offending portion of the brain and is then connected to an impulse generator. The patient is actually awake (but sedated) during the procedure so that the surgeon can monitor and modify the actions and responses of the patient. In this manner, the electrical lead can be placed with the *utmost precision* in order to avoid any unforeseen or unintended consequence—who wants to leave the hospital after surgery and wink at the first lovely lady they see only to immediately lose all bladder and bowel control? (With my kind of luck, I'm sure I would have *this* post-op complication.) Shortly after the procedure, a "pacemaker," surgically placed in the patient's upper chest, is activated and sends signals to the brain, signals that somehow aid in the transmission of the appropriate nerve impulses. Someone gets to live a more normal life.

Should you have an interest in this procedure, for yourself or for a loved one, ask your physician for a surgical referral. There is a great little video clip about the pacemaker and the procedure on YouTube. Search for it by title, or use the complicated web address below should you have trouble locating this particular video presentation.

> **—Deep Brain Stimulation an Effective Therapy for Parkinson's**
> www.king5.com/health/Deep-brain-stimulation-parkinsons-162665436.html

You are *not* going to believe this

So I won't tell you. Okay, I will tell you (because I was planning to all along). It starts from observations made with respect to MS. MS has a lot of enemies, including Dr. D. Craig Hooper. He is a scientist who is involved in studying the role played by uric acid in both health and disease—yes, the same uric acid that causes so much trouble for the person who suffers from gout. Unknown to many, uric acid plays an important role in protecting cells from damaging free radicals. Astonishingly, up to 60% of the antioxidant capability of the blood that bathes our cells is handled by this little molecule! (Boban and Modun, 2010) Certain atoms or molecules known as free radicals, unless properly dealt with, directly damage neurons as well as their surrounding myelin sheath. Uric acid binds these atoms and molecules, neutralizing them to avoid damage to healthy tissues and cells. Free radical damage is intimately involved in the pathogenesis of both MS and Parkinson's, and uric acid's job is to neutralize and limit their destructive capacity. Now this is the part that gets a little unbelievable: ***There has never been a clearly documented case of MS in a patient with gout!*** Twenty million medical records were reviewed to confirm this observation. *"The two diseases are almost mutually exclusive."* (Hooper et al., 1998) The elevated uric acid levels, as seen in gout patients, seem to protect against MS. In fact, MS patients typically have low uric acid levels, so they are missing out on its protective effects. And, yes, the same is true for patients with Parkinson's disease. The ability to increase uric acid levels by taking a supplement called inosine is being seriously considered as a formal therapy. And why inosine? Inosine breaks down into uric acid shortly after ingestion and raises the uric acid level in the bloodstream in a dose-dependent manner. This method of increasing uric acid levels is not just theory, it actually works. So it is not surprising that one of the most well-known Parkinson's patients in the universe, Michael J. Fox, has, through his foundation, donated 5.6 million dollars towards research into the use of inosine for Parkinson's disease. There is real promise here! This story can be told in the following papers:

—**Parkinson's Funded Grant**
www.michaeljfox.org/foundation/grant-detail.php?grant_id=403

—**From Gout Culprit to MS Treatment?**
http://news.sciencemag.org/sciencenow/1997/03/19-03.html

—**Hooper DC, Spitsin S, Kean RB, Champion JM, Dickson GM, Chaidhry I, Koprowski H** 1998 Uric Acid, a Natural Scavenger of Peroxynitrite, in Experimental Allergic Encephalomyelitis and Multiple Sclerosis. Proc. Natl. Acad. Sci.; January; 95:675–680

—**Weisskopf MG, O'Reilly E, Chen H, Schwartzchild MA, Ascherio A** 2007 Plasma Urate and Risk of Parkinson's Disease. American Journal of Epidemiology 166(5):561–567

Chapter 11
Alzheimer's disease (AD)

Vitamin D exhibits functional attributes that may prove neuro-protective through antioxidative mechanisms, neuronal calcium regulation, immunomodulation, enhanced nerve conduction and detoxification mechanisms. **Compelling evidence supports a beneficial role for the active form of vitamin D in the developing brain as well as in adult brain function.** **~Buell and Dawson-Hughes, 2008, emphasis added**

Associations have been noted between low 25-hydroxyvitamin D [25(OH)D] and Alzheimer's disease and dementia in both Europe and the US. Similarly, the risk of cognitive impairment was up to four times greater in the severely deficient elders (25(OH)D <25 nmol/L) in comparison with individuals with adequate levels (≥75 nmol/L). **~Soni et al., 2012**

In conclusion, vitamin D clearly has a beneficial role in AD and improves cognitive function in some patients with AD. **~Quốc Lu'o'ng and Nguyen, 2011**

S ay "Hello" to another disease to live in fear of. Alzheimer's—a disease so horrible that it, too, bears the name of a person—is certainly high on the list of dreadful diseases to avoid. It is becoming clear that hypovitaminosis D, year after year after year after year, increases your risk. And Alzheimer's is a *most* dreadful disease. It allows you the opportunity to lose your mind, but never the ability to find it. You decline on all levels. You die. *This* is the disease we call Alzheimer's. You won't like Alzheimer's, but you won't know that you don't like Alzheimer's. It's that bad.

It is believed that vitamin D sufficiency offers protection against all forms of dementia, including Alzheimer's disease. *"Low 25(OH)D concentrations may increase the risk of cerebrovascular pathology and mediate the risk of dementia via increased hypertension, diabetes, cardiovascular disease, and atherosclerosis."* (Soni et al., 2012) There's more.

Perhaps most importantly, *"1,25(OH)D$_2$D3 strongly stimulates phagocytic clearance of amyloid β (Aβ) plaques, a hallmark pathological lesion in AD which triggers neurodegeneration in primary cortical neurons."* (Soni et al., 2012) So what does this Aβ business mean? It means that the "active" vitamin D is intimately involved in a certain, vital, housekeeping activity that normally occurs within the brain. The macrophage, an immune cell that lives and works within the brain, should be "eating" these Aβ plaques for lunch by a process called phagocytosis. But apparently, less of this occurs when vitamin D supplies are low. The Aβ formations that are normally produced are not cleared as intended. As they accumulate, the transmission of nerve impulses are blocked, the function of the brain declines (Ito et al., 2011), and, as a bonus, you get to hide your own Easter eggs.

Vitamin D performs a number of important tasks that ease the effects of aging on the brain. Vitamin D, by its anti-inflammatory actions, reduces the burden of systemic low-grade inflammation as well as inflammation that somehow rises up within the brain itself, both of which are harmful to its health and function (Holmes et al., 2009; Quốc Lu'o'ng et al., 2011). Vitamin D protects against free radical damage within the brain (and elsewhere) by enhancing antioxidant defenses (Soni et al., 2012). Vitamin D is also essential for vascular health everywhere including the brain (Annweiler et al., 2011). Since evidence exists that *"vascular dysfunction plays an important role in early progression of AD,"* it is anticipated that vitamin D sufficiency will help protect against Alzheimer's disease and other forms of dementia by promoting cerebrovascular health (Ito et al., 2011). Therefore, in the setting of hypovitaminosis D day after day after day after day, cerebrovascular disease is more likely to develop and progress, making dementia and Alzheimer's disease more likely to occur. Of course, cerebrovascular disease limits the flow of oxygen and nutrients to areas of the brain, important areas. All things considered, is it any wonder that the risk of dementia and Alzheimer's increase in the setting of hypovitaminosis D? Is it any wonder that I want you to pay close attention to the following two quotations?

> A significant association between severe 25(OH)D3 deficiency <10 ng/ml and advanced-stage dementia was found among 288 elderly inpatients aged 86 years on average, regardless of the type of dementia. In line with this result, a **2.2 fold increased risk of dementia** was also shown among community-dwellers with hypovitaminosis D. (Annweiler et al., 2011, emphasis added)

> Analysis of data from older people referred to a US geriatric outpatient clinic with a diagnosis of probable Alzheimer's disease demonstrated a significant association between vitamin D deficiency and cognitive impairment. In a US community sample, those with severe deficiency (<25 nmol/L) were **four times as likely to be cognitively impaired** compared with those with serum levels of ≥75 nmol/L. (Dickens et al., 2011, emphasis added)

Okay, I think I have made my point. **You ... have ... been ... warned!** Vitamin D deficiency day after day after day after day increases your risk of dementia, including the dreadful disease called Alzheimer's. Perhaps vitamin D deficiency, day after day after day after day (and day after day after day), will not serve the dementia patient well. In order to prevent Alzheimer's disease and other forms of dementia, it seems reasonable to achieve and maintain a respectable degree of vitamin D sufficiency. So is it any wonder that I have added cognitive decline, dementia, and Alzheimer's disease to my list of reasons to achieve vitamin D sufficiency and remain sufficient for life? Does *this* sound like fun to you?

> The majority of people with dementia exhibit clinically significant neuropsychiatric symptoms, and in the latter stages dementia results in total dependency, frailty and death. The impact on families can be devastating and caregiving is associated with substantial psychological and physical morbidity. (Dickens et al., 2011)

Extra credit

If you wish to learn a little more about Alzheimer's, I have a great little slide show for you to watch, well done and very informative. It is produced by the *Alzheimer's Association*. Type **alz.org/braintour** in the search box of your browser to locate this presentation, or you can use the web address given below.

—Braintour
www.alz.org/braintour/3_main_parts.asp

Not again!

> *Body iron stores that increase with age could be pivotal to AD pathogenesis and progression. Increased stored iron is associated with common medical conditions such as diabetes and vascular disease that increase risk for developing AD.* **~Dwyer et al., 2009**

So, once again, I issue a warning about iron (but you don't seem to be listening). Iron is intimately involved in the disease process known as Alzheimer's. Pay attention! Iron intake, in excess of individual need, has the capacity to challenge and damage cells, brain cells included. It accumulates day after day after day in our tissues. Add a dreadful disease process to the mix, and the threat is compounded. Iron excess and dysregulation are part of the devastation that is occurring within the Alzheimer's brain. Phlebotomy (think blood donation) may be particularly useful as a therapy to prevent further damage and improve cognition in those who suffer from Alzheimer's disease (Dwyer et al., 2009). I have added protecting my brain (or what's left of it) to the list of reasons why I regularly donate blood—when I donate blood, I donate iron. I also limit my iron intake from dietary sources, within reason. (You're not taking iron supplements without clear indication and physician approval, are you?) The following paper, written for the layperson, tells this important story. Search for it by title or by the web address listed below.

—**Excess Iron and Brain Degeneration: The Little-Known Link.**
www.lef.org/magazine/mag2012/mar2012_Excess-Iron-Brain-
Degeneration_01.htm

Chapter 12
Infectious disease

Vitamin D deficiency has long been correlated with a high incidence of infection, suggesting that this deficiency may enhance susceptibility to infection. **~Hayes et al., 2003**

The immune system is able to distinguish between foreign invaders (bacteria and viruses) and the "self" body tissues in normal, healthy individuals. **~Cantorna, 2000**

In wound repair, 1,25(OH)$_2$D$_3$ enables keratinocytes [the predominate skin cell type] to protect against infection, and highlight that this hormone is a key component of innate immunity in the antimicrobial response following injury. **~Adorini and Penna, 2008**

Antimicrobial peptides [e.g., cathelicidin] are part of the innate immune system of many species and are thought to provide protection against bacteria, fungi, and viruses, either by directly killing or binding to bacterial endotoxin and blunting the biological effects of infection. **~Bals et al., 1999**

African American women receiving 2,000 IU of vitamin D$_3$ /d [per day] had a 93% reduction in reported upper respiratory tract infections. **~Holick, 2008**

To be disease resistant from an infectious-disease standpoint, you need to live in a "bubble" or you need a strong, sophisticated immune system (like the one I have). It's your choice! Just so you know, a bubble is only fun for about 4 minutes. Then the loneliness sets in.

The research is abundantly clear: We need sunlight exposure, *"the primary determinate of vitamin D status in humans"* (Ginde et al., 2009), or we need Plan B done *exceptionally well*—particularly during winter— to adequately protect us from a variety of infectious diseases. And there are *so* many to choose from. Take your pick! And it's not just a healthy immune system that is necessary to prevent infection; it is the production of certain molecules, molecules produced, no doubt, by genetic programs that also get in on the act. One such molecule is called cathelicidin (I know, "Never heard of it!"). The production of this molecule (also called LL37) is related to the vitamin D status of the individual. If vitamin D levels are low, cathlicidin production will be low and the risk for infection will be elevated. So let's take a minute and look at this little game-changer.

Cathelicidin is an antimicrobial protein secreted by a wide variety of cells, particularly by surface cells such as the skin (Adorini and Penna, 2008; Segaert and Simonart, 2008), the mucous membranes (Bals et al., 1999), the cells that form the lining of the bowel (Schmidt and Mangelsdorf, 2008), as well as the cells that line the respiratory tract (Bals et al., 1999). If a cell goes to the trouble to produce it, it is probably important. And it is not just surface cells that produce cathelicidin; various cells of our immune system also produce and release this molecule. It is actually "blood in the water" for migratory immune cells, attracting them, like sharks, to their next feeding frenzy (Adorini and Penna, 2008; Hata et al., 2008; Ginde et al., 2009). Cathelicidin serves as one of our initial defenses against foreign invaders. It can kill directly or it can enhance the killing ability of certain immune cells that arrive on the scene to do battle (Schmidt and Mangelsdorf, 2008). Cathelicidin production is *dramatically* increased by vitamin D, and this response against infection is *greatly* weakened when vitamin D is in short supply (Hata, 2008; Ginde et al., 2009). Who knows how much trouble is prevented when the production of this antimicrobial is unimpaired? Who knows? Pneumonia is trouble. TB is trouble. Influenza is trouble. The common cold is trouble. Strep throat is trouble. Paracoccidioidomycosis is trouble. I could go on and on about trouble. And I will. I am *not* about to stop, not when the health of the unborn is at stake!

It has been clearly demonstrated that vitamin D deficiency in the mother-to-be may invite infectious organisms to enter, threaten, and compromise the life of the one who is developing inside. Bacterial infection in the mother-to-be can lead to fetal demise, in addition to a wide variety of health problems that become evident soon after birth or later in life (Grayson and Hewison, 2011). The vaginal production of cathelicidin can help reduce this threat to the unborn. And, as a backup, the placenta also produces this antimicrobial in order to protect the one developing inside from game-changing infectious disease (Grayson and Hewison, 2011). Mothers-to-be who are deficient in vitamin D—therefore deficient in cathelicidin—are placing their unborn babies at increased risk of some very bad things.

How do we pull this off?

Fighting infection is quite a feat. And the ability to ward off attack is required 24/7, or we die! The body has many defense mechanisms, along with a whole host of specialized cells that silently protect us from harm. When the time comes to mount a fierce battle, we have the tools for this, too. And, not only does our immune system defend us, it also promotes tissue repair after the battle subsides. The following video gives us a glimpse of some of the actions that our immune system takes in order to keep us around. There is not a day that goes by that I do not thank my lucky stars for my extremely sophisticated and very cool immune system. (Okay, I forget from time to time.) Search for the following, watch, and be amazed!

—**Acute Inflammation 2009**
www.youtube.com/watch?v=suCKm97yvyk

The flu (and you)

Historically, the flu has been quite costly in terms of human life. For example, in 1918 a flu epidemic took the lives of between 50 and 100 million people. (I still miss them.) Even today, the flu kills an estimated 250,000 to 500,000 individuals each year! It appears that vitamin D deficiency will increase the risk of contracting the flu. It may even contribute to its severity.

Characteristically, flu season is a phenomenon that occurs during the low-vitamin D-availability months of winter, prompting this statement: *"Compelling epidemiological evidence indicates vitamin D deficiency is the 'seasonal stimulus.'"* (Cannell et al., 2008) When you have the flu, you are going to have to eat (phagocytose) the little buggers that have invaded. (Or you die!) Fortunately, we have a cell for that. The macrophage will do this for you free of charge, but it will need a little help. *"Phagocytic function of human macrophages is enhanced in individuals who receive vitamin D supplementation."* (Heaney, 2008) It seems a little shortsighted to push for flu vaccination in our population while, at the same time, we pay little if any attention to vitamin D. But then again, we do live in a crazy world. Unfortunately, the flu is particularly rough on our elderly population. Unfortunately, vitamin D deficiency in the elderly is almost universal, with the exception of those who supplement in relevant amounts.

To see how a flu virus is transmitted and how it infects the host, watch the following video. It is quite a video, very fascinating and exceptionally well done. You should watch this instead of one of your dumb TV shows.

—Flu Attack! How A Virus Invades Your Body
www.youtube.com/watch?v=Rpj0emEGShQ&feature

Chapter 13
Cardiovascular disease

Living at higher latitude and vitamin deficiency are also associated with hypertension and cardiovascular disease. Li et al. reported that 1,25(OH)$_2$D$_3$ is an effective regulator of rennin production, which controls blood pressure. **~Holick, 2006**

A recent study has brought forward evidence that a low vitamin D status also contributes to the pathogenesis of congestive heart failure, a disease resulting in cardiac muscle weakness due to impaired myocardial contractility.

Low vitamin D status can explain alterations in mineral metabolism as well as myocardial dysfunction in the CHF [congestive heart failure] patients, and it may therefore be a contributing factor in the pathogenesis of CHF.

Interestingly, vitamin D plays a pivotal role in cardiac function. Cardiac muscle cells possess a vitamin D receptor and a calcitriol-dependent Ca^{2+} binding protein. Moreover, a calcitriol-mediated rapid activation of voltage-dependent Ca^{2+} channels exists in cardiac muscle cells. **~Zittermann et al., 2003**

Vitamin D deficiency and/or increased PTH levels also predisposes to calcification of heart valves, mitral annulus, and myocardium, especially in patients with moderate to severe chronic kidney disease. **~Lee et al., 2008**

Low levels of 25(OH)D and 1,25-dihydroxyvitamin D are associated with prevalent myocardial dysfunction, deaths due to heart failure, and SCD [sudden cardiac death]. **~Pilz et al., 2008**

Taken together, the preceding series of quotations tell a compelling story, a story of a close relationship between vitamin D and the cardiovascular health. It sounds like people could get into a lot of trouble should their vitamin D status be compromised and remain unaddressed. Cardiovascular disease is trouble, big trouble!

One study of 1,739 people, people who were free of cardiovascular disease at the beginning of the study, found a **53% to 80%** higher chance of fatal and non-fatal heart attacks, ischemia, stroke, or heart failure if the study participant was vitamin D deficient (Lee et al., 2008). And no one—**no one!**—not even the physician, is safe. *"A study of male health professionals showed a **2-fold risk** of myocardial infarction (MI) in subjects who were vitamin D deficient compared with those in the sufficient range."* (Lee et al., 2008, emphasis added)

I guess the lesson here is that the effects of vitamin D deficiency are so pervasive that nothing is **sacred**, not even the **heart**. (What a coincidence! I work at a hospital named ***Sacred Heart.***) Vitamin D deficiency not only affects the performance of the heart, related to the role vitamin D plays in the regulation of intracellular calcium (Zittermann et al., 2003), but it also contributes to many if not most of the risk factors associated with disease of the heart.

The effect of vitamin D insufficiency will probably not be noticed until the heart is compromised by other factors, but the research suggests (very impressively, may I add) that hypovitaminosis D is playing a silent but deadly role.

The heart of the matter is this: The heart needs vitamin D, both directly and indirectly, in order to continue to proudly serve. (I would say pumping 1,900 gallons of blood per day is proudly serving.) In addition, our vasculature—some 60,000 to 100,000 miles in length, including the arteries that feed the heart muscle itself—is comprised of cells that need vitamin D in adequate amounts in order to stay elastic and stay healthy. Of course, we should include the risk of stroke in our little discussion of vitamin D and cardiovascular health.

Stroke typically occurs as a consequence of vascular disease. So it should come as no surprise that stroke is simply more prevalent in those who are vitamin D deficient (Lee et al., 2008; Balden et al., 2012). Actually death is more prevalent in those who are vitamin D deficient. But you don't have to die to be a victim of vitamin D deficiency.

> Vitamin D deficiency seems to predispose to hypertension, diabetes, and the metabolic syndrome, left ventricular hypertrophy, congestive heart failure, and chronic vascular inflammation. (Lee et al., 2008)

Furthermore,

> Vitamin D and calcium are independently and interactively involved in many pathophysiologic processes related to the development of CVD [cardiovascular disease]. Vitamin D downregulates the rennin-angiotension system [involved in hypertension], improves insulin secretion and sensitivity, inhibits vascular smooth-muscle cell proliferation, protects normal endothelial cell function, and modulates inflammatory processes. Epidemiologic studies have found an association between vitamin D insufficiency, reflected by low serum 25-dyhydroxyvitamin D levels, and higher rates of CVD morbidity. (Wang et al., 2010)

And since mention was made of calcium, don't forget to remember this:

> Calcium supplements (without coadministration with vitamin D) are associated with an increased risk of myocardial infarction. (Bolland et al., 2010)

With our little discussion of cardiovascular health and vitamin D now out of the way, it may be safe to move on to the next chapter. Maybe. But before we move on (in fear and trepidation), I do have a little more related information I would like to share.

Cardiac disease unplugged

I will forgo the reverences here. I simply want to tell you a little story. We'll go back in time, say, a little over 100 years ago.

Around the beginning of the 20th century—and my sources tell me that this is true—a world-famous physician named Sir William Osler had just published a comprehensive textbook on medicine. When asked why he left out a chapter on heart disease, he stated: "Heart disease is so rare; I don't think the average physician will ever see it!" Interestingly enough, this was a time in our history when we ate freely of saturated fat and couldn't care less about cholesterol. The point here is this: Once, in the not-too-distant past, heart disease—even heart attack—was relatively uncommon. This is quite surprising, given the rate of heart disease today and the fact that our genetics are no different today than they were 100 years ago. My, how times have changed! Heart disease is now our number-one killer! And I've seen this killer at work. I, personally, have spent nearly a quarter of a century recovering open heart surgery patients immediately post op, in addition to taking care of patients who have acutely suffered a heart attack—and the cardiac patients I have cared for over the years number in the thousands! So I do know, firsthand, how prevalent heart disease is today. Why the change over the course of a single century? Let's take a look.

During the past 100 years, remarkable changes occurred in our diet, changes that our genes were simply not ready to handle. Perhaps most significantly, we dramatically altered the fatty acid composition in our diet. Today we consume what should be considered an "extreme" amount of the proinflammatory omega-6 fatty acids, day in and day out, and think nothing of it. In addition, trans fats, artificially created, entered our food supply and began the task of destroying life. But there is more to consider.

During this same period of time—and particularly during the past 60 years or so—inexpensive, high-calorie, processed "junk" foods began to arrive on the scene in ever increasing amounts (typically high in the omega-6 fatty acids). In response, our diet evolved into what we now call the *Western diet*. Say "Hello" to the insulin resistance syndrome, otherwise known as the metabolic syndrome. And, to add insult to injury, smoking arrived on the scene, enslaved many, and began the task of destroying a large portion of our population. Smoking is and remains a huge risk factor for cardiac disease—even secondhand smoking is not without risk in this regard. But there was more trouble ahead for our society. And I do mean trouble.

Over the past 50-plus years, added to the Western diet were increasing amounts of fructose, the tasty little molecule found in table sugar and high-fructose corn syrup. The consumption of fructose <u>from any source</u>, above a certain threshold, strongly contributes to the risk factors for coronary artery disease, and particularly contributes to our alarming rate of obesity and diabetes. *"There is strong evidence that diets high in fructose can produce obesity, insulin resistance/glucose intolerance, and dyslipidemia."* (Stanhope and Havel, 2008)

And in the background of all of the above was this thing called vitamin D deficiency, playing a subtle yet deadly role.

Of course, there is more to the story, as there is with any story. But I have given you the highlights. If you are a smoker, you need to seriously consider quitting. If you're an eater, seriously consider eating more healthfully. Eating more healthfully used to mean <u>drastically</u> limiting the saturated fats, but not anymore. We now know better. Eating more healthfully means avoiding artificially produced trans fats and <u>drastically</u> limiting the omega-6 fatty acids, as found in the snack and convenience foods, the fried foods, the salad dressings, the vegetable cooking oils (like safflower, sunflower, corn, and soybean oils), and the vegetable margarines. But there is one more problem that needs to be addressed, one that undoubtedly accelerates the development of cardiovascular disease in one hungry individual at a time. It is this fructose molecule mentioned above. Later, I will give you a video series to watch related to the dangers of fructose. I will tack it on to my chapter on obesity.

More to the story

The following is not what you have been told. You have been told that saturated fat is certainly out to kill you. But it wasn't out to kill you a hundred years ago! Carefully consider this:

> In early 20th century Britain and the United States everyone cooked and baked with butter or lard, and death from what we now call myocardial infarction was so rare that it had no name or medical recognition. The oilseed industry was founded shortly before 1920 and by 1926 was injecting into the national diet trainloads of new vegetable fats which, in the concept of the "prudent" diet are now the "good" fats . . . I suggest that the introduction of *trans- trans* linoleic acid in the 1920s in margarines and refined vegetable oils was the main cause of the pandemic of myocardial infarction and that since 1960 orthodox medicine has been fostering a cause of this disease as the cure. (MacDonald, 2008, quoting Dr. Wayne Martin)

Strangely enough, it is the introduction of the omega-6 seed oils, in ever-increasing amounts, that has introduced us to our number one-killer. Ignoring this issue is costing lives. Today, many cultures consume, by our standards, large amounts of saturated fat including cholesterol. And, paradoxically, they have much lower rates of cardiovascular disease. I thought you would like to know this, even though it goes against conventional thought. You're eating saturated fat anyway, so you might as well not feel so much guilt over it. But don't overdo it here! I want you to save room for other healthy fatty acids, like the monounsaturated fatty acids from avocado and olive oil, like the medium-chain fatty acids from coconut and real butter, and like the omega-3 fatty acids found in fish and dark green leafy vegetables. Of course, should you receive a recommendation from your physician to limit your intake of saturated fat (and cholesterol), you should follow this advice. Once a disease process is established, the dos and don'ts typically change.

Chapter 14
Neurodevelopmental and psychiatric disorders

Profound alterations in the brain at birth have been demonstrated in rats born to vitamin D deficient mothers. **~VanAmerongen et al., 2004, emphasis added**

Epidemiological study of other disease processes that raise the possibility for positive association with maternal vitamin D status in pregnancy includes osteoporosis, multiple sclerosis, and schizophrenia. **~Taylor et al., 2009**

Living at higher latitudes increases the risk of schizophrenia. **~Holick, 2008**

Animal data has repeatedly shown that severe vitamin D deficiency during gestation dysregulates dozens of proteins involved in brain development and leads to rat pups with increased brain size and enlarged ventricles, abnormalities similar to those found in autistic children. **~Cannell, 2008**

Remember your life as a mouse in *Chapter 8*? *That* did not go well! (Although your twin is doing just fine and having lots of fun.) Well, over the years you have changed a little and have packed on some weight—now you are one big rat! And, again, things are definitely not going your way! You will now be the focus of an experiment to see if you can come down with the same physiologic features found in autism and schizophrenia patients. Your outlook looks grim, very grim. I see an autopsy in your future. (I will probably not be asked to be a fortune cookie writer.)

No, I'm not making any of this up! They, the scientists, have noticed a few things that are not quite right in the brains of autistic and schizophrenic patients. The brain cavities and structures of those affected are malformed in various degrees (Eyles et al., 2007; Féron et al., 2005; Cannell, 2008). In addition, a substantial degree of dysregulation in brain chemistry occurs in both of these medical conditions (Eyles et al., 2007; Cannell, 2008). It is quite remarkable that they, the scientists (perhaps mad scientists?), can produce the same identical, __*profound*__ changes in rat offspring that occur in the patients with autism and schizophrenia simply by making their mother significantly deficient in vitamin D during her pregnancy (Eyles et al., 2007; Cannell, 2008). That's all that it takes. What a coincidence! People can become significantly deficient in vitamin D during pregnancy, too, and can do so all on their own! Have you heard of *burkas*? Have you heard of *the night shift*? Have you heard of *sunscreen*? Have you heard of *mothers who are confined to bed during the latter part of their pregnancy*? Have you heard of *drugs* and *chemicals* that interfere with the absorption or the unitization of vitamin D? Have you heard of *smoking*? Have you heard of . . .

So, when it comes to the unborn, not only does vitamin D deficiency negatively influence brain chemistry, it can negatively alter brain architecture during gestation. Furthermore, vitamin D deficiency can also influence the quality of brain development, even after birth! Vitamin D is <u>clearly</u> a developmental hormone. *Clearly!* Nerve growth, cell differentiation, and cell survival are all regulated, in part, by vitamin D (Llewellyn et al., 2009). It should be in adequate supply.

Now this is where things get very, very sad: Our lack of attention to the vitamin D status of the mother-to-be, and, by extension, to the one who is developing inside, can have <u>serious</u> consequences. Do you know (and love) someone who suffers from autism? Do you know (and avoid) someone who suffers from schizophrenia? For this lack of attention to vitamin D, we as a society, and those negatively affected, are paying a huge price. I just have to point out the following: The use of sunscreen in our society has certainly not helped—*its progressive use parallels the increase in the incidence of autism!* (Cannell, 2008) Coincidence? I doubt it. Then there is schizophrenia.

> Both low and high concentrations of neonatal vitamin D are associated with increased risk of schizophrenia, and it is feasible that this exposure could contribute to a sizable proportion of cases in Denmark. In light of the substantial public health implications of this finding, there is an urgent need to further explore the effect of vitamin D status on brain development and later mental health. (McGrath et al., 2010)

The association between vitamin D deficiency and the risk of schizophrenia is underscored by the fact that migrating populations of people who are dark skinned and have moved from a sunny region like Somalia to a "sunlight-impaired" region like northern Europe experience a significant increase in the incidence of schizophrenia in their offspring (McGrath, 2001; Cannel, 2008). Coincidence? I doubt it.

You did not know any of this, so stop pretending. Go, get your vitamin D level checked before you take whatever steps are required in order to make a baby. (I'm trying to remember what the steps are.) Your responsibility starts well before the pregnancy begins. At the very least, once you are aware that you are pregnant, be sure to get your vitamin D level checked—the glow that comes along with pregnancy will not be bright enough to provide you or your baby with any vitamin D. Of course I am talking to the ladies here, but you gentlemen can be aware of the issues, too, and can insist that vitamin D deficiency be screened for and corrected. You want a healthy baby, too, right? Besides, some couples can never become pregnant or maintain pregnancy should the ladies' hypovitaminosis D go unidentified and unresolved.

Before we leave this section, please consider this: It is well known that mental health requires a normal, functioning synapse, and a neurotransmitter economy that works as intended. Many psychiatric medications target the synapse and facilitate neurotransmission. Well, so does vitamin D! (Garcion et al., 2002; Eyles et al., 2003; Eyles et al., 2007; McCann and Ames, 2008) Even the architectural development of the synapse itself is regulated by vitamin D (Eyles et al., 2007; Cannell, 2008; Fernandes de Abreu et al., 2009). Yet this vitamin, this hormone, is too often ignored in the treatment of both psychological and neurological disorders. Sounds crazy to me! (It is about to drive me nuts.)

No one in their right mind would write a chapter on psychiatric disorders without at least a short discussion on depression and vitamin D deficiency. Depression is so out there, and so treated with anything but vitamin D that this, too, is about to drive me . . . well you know. Even though the following is a bit heavy on the science, you will get the idea that vitamin D could play a very important role in the prevention and treatment of depression.

> Vitamin D is a unique neurosteroid hormone that may have an important role in the development of depression. Receptors for vitamin D are present on neurons and glia in many areas of the brain including the cingulate cortex and hippocampus, which have been implicated in the pathophysiology of depression. Vitamin D is involved in numerous brain processes including neuroimmuno-modulation, regulation of neurotrophic factors, neuroprotection, neuroplasticity and brain development, making it biologically plausible that this vitamin might be associated with depression and that its supplementation might play an important part in the treatment of depression. (Anglin et al., 2013)

Yes, I have another book

Let me tell you about another book I wrote. It is entitled *Preventing Birth Defects: Understanding the Thyroid Hormone Connection*. And why would I write such a book? It's kind of a long story, but I'll be brief.

I first started avidly (relentlessly) reading medical journals roughly 15 years ago, all in an effort to understand the subtleties of hypothyroidism. This quest <u>consumed</u> several years of my life. And what do I have to show for it? A little paper called *Hypothyroidism Redefined*. I am very proud of this paper and have made it available on my website. It strongly suggests that we take a different approach to the treatment of this disease and outlines an alternative. But what I am most proud of is the book that this study spawned (spawned is a reproductive term, in case you were not paying attention).

During my comprehensive study of hypothyroidism, I stumbled across a story the layperson is basically unaware of and the medical community is, quite frankly, not paying close enough attention to. Yet it is a story of profound significance. Compelled to bring the issues involved to the forefront, I carefully developed, then placed in book form perhaps one of the most important stories that can be told about the prevention of birth defects. In the book I speak of iodine and how iodine deficiency negatively impacts fetal development. I also speak of careful screening for hypothyroidism and related disorders, in addition to careful screening for iodine deficiency, in order to insure that the unborn individual does not enter this world damaged and beyond repair. We're talkin' the *major* birth defects associated with hypothyroidism and iodine deficiency like cerebral palsy, mental retardation, cardiac defects, psychiatric disorders, and other serious problems that can have their beginnings, sometimes, even before the mother-to-be knows she is pregnant. We can end so much tragedy and sadness by paying <u>close</u> attention to the thyroid and iodine status of ladies who make babies. None of this is all that difficult, and by taking appropriate action many individuals can be spared from a life of great challenge and spared of no life at all. But don't take my word for it (although you should probably start doing this); you can take the word of these two physicians.

Iodine deficiency increases neonatal mortality. **We emphasize this statement so that iodine deficiency can take its proper place among disorders that kill children.**

Iodine deficiency poses additional reproductive risks, including overt hypothyroidism, infertility, and increased abortions. Hypothyroidism causes anovulation, infertility, gestational hypertension, increased first trimester abortions, and stillbirths: all are common in iodine deficiency.

The most vulnerable target for iodine deficiency is the developing brain. Iodine is critical to maturation of the central nervous system.

Mental retardation from iodine deficiency is not limited to the extreme form of cretinism, but instead extends over a broad continuum to mild intellectual blunting that may go unrecognized unless carefully investigated. Thus, iodine deficiency puts virtually everyone in the affected population at some risk for brain damage. (Dunn and Delange, 2001, emphasis added)

Did you know any of this? Does your daughter know any of this? Does your health care provider routinely perform <u>careful</u> screening, including screening for iodine deficiency, subclinical hypothyroidism, and antithyroid antibodies on <u>everyone</u> who is pregnant or likely to become pregnant? I can't think of a more important story to tell. *I can't!* If corrective action is taken at the very beginning of a pregnancy (especially before), so much evil can be prevented. Sadly, in the USA one in one hundred babies is born with a serious birth defect. We should try our best to put a dent into this statistic. But so often, we leave things to chance . . . and hope for the best.

Preventing Birth Defects: Understanding the Thyroid Hormone Connection is now available from my website and on Amazon.com. What a wonderful gift it would be for someone whose desire it is to provide the best start in life for the brand new little person she will be creating. This book will change everything! (If all goes as planned.)

Chapter 15
Muscles and bones

There is general agreement that low vitamin D status is involved in the pathogenesis of osteoporosis. Moreover, vitamin D insufficiency can lead to a disturbed muscle function. **~Zittermann, 2003**

If the vitamin D input never becomes low enough to produce clinical rickets, then its deficiency is expressed solely as osteoporosis. **~Heaney, 2003**

So, on one side severe vitamin D deficiency causes a mineralization problem and osteomalacia and on the other side the high PTH [parathyroid hormone] levels cause high bone turnover, bone resorption and osteoporosis and both mechanisms may lead to fractures, especially hip fractures. **~Lips, 2006**

Osteomalacia due to vitamin D depletion appears not to be suspected or diagnosed promptly in susceptible patients, perhaps because their physicians were not sufficiently aware of this condition.

We have observed a <u>general lack of awareness</u> about osteomalacia among clinicians. **~Basha et al., 2000, emphasis added**

Consequently, very low 25(OH)D levels as found in rickets and osteomalacia results in an impaired intestinal Ca [calcium] absorption leading to severe Ca deficit in the human body.

There is, however, also evidence that 25(OH)D levels below 25 nmol/l can lead to rickets and osteomalacia in the long run.

Patients with osteomalacia suffer from muscle weakness and have low serum levels of muscle enzymes. **~Zittermann, 2003**

This chapter touches briefly on the importance of normal skeletal remodeling and normal muscle function—both being clearly under the regulatory influence of vitamin D. And, of course, calcium is intimately involved. In a low vitamin D state, bone remodeling is compromised. And, perhaps, at the same time, bad things happen to muscle.

At this very moment, your bones are continually being remodeled, torn apart, yet, at the same time, being rebuilt in order to maintain bone strength and deal with calcium loss. Leave it to the vitamin D hormone to take an active role in this normal remodeling process. (Let's hope it is in adequate supply.) What is surprising is, even in the face of low vitamin D levels, bone remodeling can be positively influenced simply by increasing an individual's calcium intake (Sutton and MacDonald, 2003). But, as we have previously discussed, high calcium consumption, in the face of hypovitaminosis D, can contribute to the risk of cardiovascular disease (Bolland et al., 2010). You probably don't want cardiovascular disease any time soon. And you certainly don't want your bones to fall apart as you get older. So take heed, and don't forget to add vitamin D, in relevant amounts, when supplementing with calcium. A "relevant amount" of vitamin D is certainly more than what you will find in a multivitamin, certainly more than is found in a combination calcium/vitamin D supplement, perhaps even more than the 1,000–2,000 IU/d recommendation that is common today. It will take a blood test to find this out for the particular individual. And you may not even need as much calcium supplementation as currently recommended. Let me explain.

The ability to absorb calcium can be increased by as much as 50% in the presence of an adequate vitamin D level (Lee et al., 2008). Therefore, less calcium consumption will be required when vitamin D levels are sufficient.

Aside from the task of favoring the absorption of calcium, vitamin D has a *direct* influence on the cells intimately involved in the remodeling process, so you get to have stronger bones, bones that will not fall apart later in life (Haussler et al., 2008; Takasu, 2008). But there is a lot more to the story. Without an adequate level of vitamin D, not only can we damage bone, we can negatively impact muscle. Skeletal muscle strength can be appreciably diminished in the setting of vitamin D deficiency, and, over time, an often-overlooked medical condition called osteomalacia may develop.

Today, while all the focus seems to be on osteoporosis—its prevention, its treatment—another bone disease, osteomalacia, frequently occurs and goes unnoticed (Basha et al., 2000; Holick, 2006a). You may have never heard of it before. On both x-ray and bone densitometry, osteoporosis and osteomalacia look the same (Holick, 2002; Holick, 2008). Unfortunately, the patient presenting with aches and pains is often given the diagnosis of fibromyalgia rather than osteomalacia. Again, a misdiagnosis is made, and the muscle aches and pains will not be properly addressed. This happens all too frequently. Let's talk a little more about osteomalacia.

Osteomalacia

The disease, osteomalacia, is called *"adult rickets"* (Holick, 2002) and is one very painful disease (Holick, 2006b). What seems to be occurring in osteomalacia is this: In the absence of adequate vitamin D, a remodeling bone cell called the osteoblast deposits a collagen matrix that should be home to new calcium deposits. Instead of receiving a new deposit of calcium, as intended, the matrix sits there and waits for something favorable to happen. While it waits, instead of being properly mineralized, the collagen matrix progressively hydrates and becomes weak and rubbery (Holick, 2003; Mascarenhas and Mobarhan, 2994). When hydration of the collagen matrix transpires—and it will— swelling will occur and place pressure on an array of regional sensory nerves, giving rise to pain. The pain of osteomalacia is often described as a *"throbbing, aching pain"* (Holick, 2007) or *"a dull unrelenting aching sensation"* in the bones (Holick, 2003) being often misdiagnosed as fibromyalgia (Holick, 2004b; Holick 2006b). It is commonplace to see osteomalacia being inappropriately treated with drugs that suppress inflammation, pain killers, or drugs that, in some fashion, manipulate the nervous system in an effort to deal with the symptoms.

Osteomalacia is believed to be rare and basically found only in the chronically ill, but this is clearly not the case. It is *very* common! It is simply not recognized for what it is. So much harm is caused when osteomalacia is not identified and is allowed to continue and to progress. If you are given the diagnosis of fibromyalgia, a condition affecting over 3 million people in the U.S., there is a high probability that you have osteomalacia instead (or, perhaps, in addition). If your osteomalacia continues to remain undiagnosed and is not effectively treated by aggressive calcium and vitamin D repletion, *"irreparable bone loss"* will occur (Basha et al., 2000). You don't need any more trouble. You are already a mess. In the next chapter you will learn of a simple test for osteomalacia, one that you can perform yourself.

Vitamin D analogues, best for osteoporosis and osteomalacia?

I'm convinced! I've read the studies! It seems that once the damage is done to muscle and bone, regular vitamin D may not be as helpful as an "engineered" form of vitamin D called a vitamin D analog. A vitamin D analog works in some situations simply because it does not need as much metabolic transformation in order to work its magic, or because it has the ability to create a special effect not typical of vitamin D in its "active" form. In so many diseases, it seems that various degrees of inflammation are playing a silent, subtle role—a situation that may be interfering with the proper metabolism of vitamin D. The good news is that vitamin D analogues may do the trick. The bad news: Vitamin D analogues, particularly Alfacalcidol—an analog showing great promise in the treatment of osteomalacia—are not currently available in the United States. Perhaps if we were to pay more attention to osteomalacia, there would be more awareness of the benefits offered by this vitamin D analog in the treatment of this disease. Alfacalcidol is actually an over-the-counter medication in Canada, and perhaps a few other countries, so one would think that, in the United States, it would at least be available by prescription. But, alas, it is not. But it should be. But it is not. But it should be. (Excuse me for a moment while I go and bang my head against the wall.)

The following papers are important discussions on the benefits of vitamin D analogues:

—**Schacht E, et al** 2005 The Therapeutic Effects of Alfacalcidol on Bone Strength, Muscle Metabolism and Prevention of Falls and Fractures. J Musculoskelet Neuronal Interact 5(3):273–284

—*****Scharla SH, et al** 2005 Alfacalcidol Versus Plain Vitamin D in Inflammation Induced Bone Loss. The Journal of Rheumatology 32(Suppl 76):26–32

—**Brown AJ** 2001 Therapeutic Uses of Vitamin D Analogues. American Journal of Kidney Diseases 38(5) (Suppl 5):S3–S19

—*****Lau K-H, Baylink DJ** 1999 Vitamin D Therapy of Osteoporosis: Plain Vitamin D Versus Active Vitamin D Analog (D-Hormone) Therapy. Calcif Tissue Int 65:295–306

—**Al-Badr W, Martin KJ** 2008 Vitamin D and Kidney Disease. Clin J Am Nephrol 3:1555–1560

*Not available free at this time.

Fibromyalgia story

I have spent well over a decade of my life attempting to solve the mystery of fibromyalgia, what it is, and how it selects its victims. What's my motivation? My sweet wife has it and has suffered greatly over the years from this disorder. And you think I am going to sit still and not go after this disease with all I've got?!! (You have to be joking.) After years of study, here is my conclusion: Fibromyalgia is whatever occurs that negatively affects muscles and nerves, producing, as a result, chronic widespread pain, pain that persists . . . unresolved. Well, that was pretty vague. Let's look a little deeper.

For a particular individual, fibromyalgia could simply be the symptoms of hypothyroidism, undetected or improperly managed. Hypothyroidism negatively effects just about everything, including skeletal muscle. Fibromyalgia certainly could be, as we have previously discussed, symptoms arising from prolonged vitamin D deficiency. Fibromyalgia could easily arise from any number of hormonal imbalances, particularly those related to the stress hormone cortisol. Undoubtedly, fibromyalgia could stem from a failure to adequately repair the everyday damage that occurs to muscles, damage that should be repaired at night, a time when one should be also be receiving adequate restorative sleep. This is my pet theory: Fibromyalgia could be a manifestation of insulin resistance, a state of affairs that screws up just about everything. Finally, fibromyalgia could be a subtle inflammatory response to something yet to be identified, perhaps a bacterium.

Fibromyalgia is often characterized by depression, sleeplessness, muscle pain, and more sleeplessness and more depression. (Did I mention more muscle pain?) Fibromyalgia may not be one single thing; it may be many things that are all rolled up into a ball and given a name.

Since fibromyalgia is considered to be a "modern" disease, let's see if we can give a modern person, like Betty over there, symptoms that we can later label as fibromyalgia. This should be fun! Let's get started, and do so without delay.

Of course, we will want to make Betty vitamin D deficient. That's a must! Over time, this is certain to harm muscle. And it should be fairly easy. Fortunately for us, Betty's faithful use of sunscreen has given us a good head start. Faithful sunscreen use is the gift of vitamin D deficiency.

Since Betty is a young adult and not made out of money (and neither is her husband), she will need to work. So we now find her taking a job down at the local toothbrush factory. Toothbrushes are heavy and the work is notoriously demanding, so she is only able to work part time, say, at most, 3 days a week. On the other days of the week, surrounded by all her labor-saving devices, she will make it through the day resting and watching daytime TV. Historically, Betty has never hung clothes out on a clothesline, not once in her entire life, although she thinks she has seen one on the History Channel. "The Price Is Right" and "Days of Our Lives" have become important to her, more important than going outdoors and getting a little sunshine during the time of day when she could easily make 20,000 IUs of vitamin D per session and be better protected from disease. But I did notice that she received a paltry 400 IUs of vitamin D in her multivitamin supplement this morning, so she is sure to squeak by and we may have to wait a little longer to see if the symptoms of fibromyalgia will show up. But perhaps we can speed things along. We don't have all day here.

Hey, I have an idea! Let's give her financial worries, and, just for fun, let's add the stress of pregnancy. The financial stress is sure to keep her up late at night worrying and losing sleep. And pregnancy, too, can be a very stressful event—expanding in size while being kicked at all hours by what feels like 3 pairs of legs. And what a coincidence. According to the ultrasound, Betty is expecting triplets! The pregnancy, all the kicking and all the expanding, is certain to rob Betty of good quality sleep, restorative sleep, and do so on a continual basis. Skeletal muscles do not deal well with sleep loss. We know this because muscle pain can be produced relatively quickly, even in healthy test subjects, simply by interrupting their sleep patterns. With triplets, there *will* be more sleep loss in Betty's future. Triplets are always looking for something to eat (actually, drink), on demand, day or night. But I'm getting a little ahead of my story; the triplets have not been born yet. That will soon change. After a brief 23-hour labor, they have now finally arrived on the scene.

Because Betty has been made vitamin D deficient, her breast milk will not include vitamin D. Therefore, the triplets will be sick quite often, and "Mom" will, therefore, lose even more sleep and will feel like pulling her hair out from all of the stress. (Are you able to relate to any of this?) Betty the Mom will certainly be way too tired, and far too busy, to get outdoors during the time of the day when she would directly convert sunlight into vitamin D. Goodie for us. Bad for Betty.

Now the bills are piling up, so it's back to the toothbrush factory after a brief and insufficient maternity leave. She hardly ever sees her husband anymore (he's very busy trying to get ahead in life), so we will not mention him further. But on the chance that we run into him again, Betty has asked us to scold him for not helping more around the house and helping more with the triplets, one of whom, the runt, seems to be having motor and neurodevelopmental difficulties. The doctors are stumped. Can you see that we are deliberately setting Betty up for something bad to happen? We hope that the evil will be fibromyalgia, according to our diabolical scheme. Betty, however, seems to be more resistant than expected, but we still haven't got all day. So, let's throw a few more things her way. But first . . .

Let's see where we are at. We are making sure that Betty will be low in vitamin D and will remain low for an extended period of time. We are robbing her of restorative sleep, knowing that this, too, over time, can cause a syndrome of widespread, unrelenting pain. We have made sure that the only life that she has, apart from work, is more work at home, indoors. For good measure, we have added quite a bit of stress to her life. But Betty does have an outlet (or two), offering her a little diversion from the cares of the day. It is called late-night TV.

Late-night TV has become a central feature in the little life that Betty has left (to herself). This is the time when she also does her snacking and her snuggling. Who can blame her for this? After all, she does deserve some quality time for herself and quality time with her husband. Okay, we've written him back into the story because, luckily for us (and for him), his plans include further loss of sleep for Betty. Soon after a brief period of stress relief, Betty's husband will be snoring (like a freight train), keeping Betty awake even longer and removing her further from *anything* that resembles a good night's sleep. And, poor Betty, because of her snacking on potato chips and the like, she is beginning to pack on the weight, particularly around the middle. Of course, she begins worrying about her weight and how she will fit into the bathing suit that she will never wear. All of this is according to plan. Fibromyalgia, here we come!

You and I are little stinkers. Just look what we have done to Betty! We've made her vitamin D deficient, and for an extended period of time. We've added stress, and it just keeps on coming! We have done our best to deprive her of restorative sleep. And to top it all off, we have started her down the path of living the insulin-resistant life. All the snacking (on simple carbohydrates and omega-6 fatty acids) is certain to come in handy as we inch ever closer to our goal. However, now that the triplets are all grown up, our plan may be in jeopardy. Now Betty may be able to get more sleep and have more time for leisurely outdoor activity. But don't count on it. Besides being all worn out, Betty is a creature of habit, so it is more late-night TV for her! And she will be losing even more sleep worrying over the triplets, the bills, and the possibility that the toothbrush factory will close and her job will be shipped overseas.

Now, we had nothing to do with the following, at least I don't think we did. Betty's hormones are starting to get out of whack. Things are certain to escalate! She will now become depressed (if she wasn't already). Accordingly, frequent visits will be made to her doctor, seeking relief from all her little problems. And, as luck would have it (for us), this doctor pays little attention to vitamin D, will eagerly throw drugs at symptoms, and will probably not get to the bottom of things. Betty may find some relief—drugs can be helpful—but probably not for the long haul. Her chronic vitamin D deficiency, plus everything else we have thrown at her, will eventually take its toll. The bags under her eyes, they are there for a reason.

Now the following we did not anticipate, and it is *not* good news for Betty. Betty has just found a lump in her breast. Could our devious scheme to make her vitamin D deficient, for years, have caused this unfortunate turn of events? Perhaps. But such is life.

Betty is now in a lot of trouble. Stress and worry will be intense and will dominate her life for quite some time. And bad things may happen (to muscles and precious body parts). This unfortunate turn of events may be all that it takes to push her directly into the path of fibromyalgia. I'm actually surprised that she has held out for so long with all that we have thrown her way, but we may not have to wait too much longer.

Oh! I'm so sorry! I just keep rattling on. So, to be kind to you, I will bring this story to a close. Later, I will tell you how things went for Betty (unless I forget). Besides, Betty isn't exactly a real person. But you are! And I'm a little worried about you, dear fibromyalgia patient. And my fear is that you will not receive the medical attention that you need.

But you are bright. You have learned the lessons from my story about Betty, realizing now that fibromyalgia is not the great mystery that it is made out to be. It is a disease that results from a damaging lifestyle. A drug, here, is not needed. A lifestyle change, that's what is needed! Correcting hypovitaminosis D, engaging in activities that help reduce stress (get outdoors and do stuff), making restorative sleep the highest priority, taking measures that improve insulin sensitivity, and correcting hormonal imbalances may help you walk away from this disease we call fibromyalgia, or at least give you a kinder and gentler fibromyalgia instead. Did I say walk? Walking is great form of exercise, a great way to reduce stress, and, during mid-day, a great way to get vitamin D. But start slow. You have fragile muscles at this point in time.

What a surprise! (And I didn't see it coming!) It only took one more complete paragraph for Betty to finally come down with fibromyalgia. You and I succeeded! Her doctor poked around a little, found the required number of tender spots on her neck, back, and arms, and proclaimed the news. End of story.

You will find Betty, and possibly yourself, written all over the following papers:

If you question whether fibromyalgia could result from vitamin D deficiency, read this chapter again. You should also read the following:

—**Matthana MH** 2011 The Relation between Vitamin D Deficiency and Fibromyalgia Syndrome in Women. Saudi Med J 32(9):925–929

—Biala A, Khan S, IrfanLiqbal M, Qureshi FS, Fazal MO, Shsheen M, Iqbal S 2009 Effect of vitamin D Replacement in Patients of Fibromyalgia. A.P.M.C; January–June; 3(1):51–58

If you feel the need to question whether sleep deprivation is a factor in fibromyalgia, review the following two papers:

—Moldofsky H 2008 The Significance, Assessment, and Management of Nonrestorative Sleep in Fibromyalgia Syndrome. CNS Spectr; March; 13(3) (Suppl. 5):22–26

—Dattilo M, Antunes HKM, Medeiros A, Neto AM, Souza HS, Tufik S, de Mello MT 2011 Sleep and Muscle Recovery: Endocrinological and Molecular Basis for a New and Promising Hypothesis. Medical Hypothesis 77:220–222

If you wonder if stress and hormonal imbalance is involved in fibromyalgia, read this:

—Gupta A, Silman AJ 2004 Psychological Stress and Fibromyalgia: A Review of the Evidence Suggesting a Neuroendocrine Link. Arthritis Research & Therapy 6(3):98–106

If you doubt whether insulin resistance and hyperinsulinemia is involved in fibromyalgia, I direct you to the following:

—Holmäng A, Brzeninska Z, Björntorp P 1993 Effects of Hyperinsulinemia on Muscle Fiber Composition and Capillarization. Diabetes; July; 42:1073–1081

—Mäntyselkä P, Mietola J, Niskanen L, Kumpusalo E 2008 Glucose Regulation and Chronic Pain at Multiple Sites. Rheumatology doi:10.1093/rheumatology/ken220

—Aragno A, Mastrocola R, Catalano M, Brignardello E, Danni O, Boccuzzi G 2004 Oxidative Stress Impairs Skeletal Muscle Repair in Diabetic Rats. Diatetes; April; 53:1082–1088

If you have been told that there is no muscle pathology in fibromyalgia (and you were considering believing this nonsense), you should read:

—Sprott H, Salemi S, Gay RE, Bradley LA, Alarcón GS, Oh SJ, Michel BA, Gay S 2004 Increased DNA Fragmentation and Ultrastructural Changes in Fibromyalgic Muscle Fibers. Ann Rheum Dis 63:245–251

—Gronemann ST, Ribel-Madsen S, Bartels EM, Danneskiold-Samsøe B, Bliddal H 2004 Collagen and Muscle Pathology in Fibromyalgia Patients. Rheumatology 43:27–31

—Bengtsson A 2002 The Muscle in Fibromyalgia. Rheumatology 41:721–724

The papers (all free) listed on this and the previous page can be read in less time than it takes to go to the doctor, wait in the waiting room, sit on the exam table while the doctor is trying to decide whether you are or whether you are not crazy, and the time to fill a prescription for a drug that may cause significant weight gain, further depression, and thoughts of suicide. Enough said?

I was planning to write a book on fibromyalgia. Perhaps, after writing *Fibromyalgia Story* and placing it here, I may not need to.

Chapter 16
Aches, pains, mobility

*Severe hypovitaminosis D is <u>not</u> asymptomatic. Before the clinical presentation of osteomalacia bone pain, **severe hypovitaminosis D results in a syndrome of persistent, nonspecific musculoskeletal pain.***
~Plotnikoff and Quigley, 2003, emphasis added

Skeletal muscles have receptors for $1,25(OH)_2D$, and vitamin D deficiency not only causes muscle weakness among children with rickets but also causes muscle weakness among adults with osteomalacia. Patients often complain of aching bones and muscle discomfort. Such patients are often misdiagnosed with fibromyalgia, chronic fatigue syndrome, myositis, or other nonspecific collagen vascular diseases. It is estimated that 40–60% of patients with fibromyalgia may have some component of vitamin D deficiency and osteomalacia. ~Holick, 2004

*When circulating levels of 25-hydroxyvitamin D remain chronically low (<20 nmol/l or 10 ng/ml), the skeleton is the first organ system to show overt signs of vitamin D deficiency. An early manifestation of vitamin D deficiency is called osteo-malacic myopathy. <u>**This condition is often misdiagnosed**</u> **because its symptoms are nonspecific, including diffuse muscle pain, deep bone pain, arthralgia, and parathesia, all of which lead to an alternative diagnosis such a polymyalgia, fibromyalgia, psycho-neurotic disorders ["It's all in your head!"], unspecified rheumatic disease, and malignant disease, among others.*** ~Mascarenhas and Mobarhan, 2004, emphasis added

*Up to 93% of patients with persistent pain have been reported to have hypovitaminosis D. **Furthermore, vitamin D supplementation for 3 months resulted in pain resolution in 95% of patients with chronic low back pain in one study, and after 6 months, symptom resolution . . . among women with hypovitaminosis D in another study.*** ~Atherton et al., 2009, emphasis added

Furthermore, patients with peripheral vascular disease and the common complaint of lower leg discomfort (claudication) were often found to be vitamin D deficient. The muscle weakness and pain were not due to the peripheral vascular disease but because of the vitamin D deficiency. **~Holick, 2005**

O steomalacia, *often misdiagnosed*, is just one of the painful conditions related to hypovitaminosis D. There are others. In this chapter, we will take a look at the aches and pains associated with a chronic lack of vitamin D. We will also take a look at the mobility issues that show up and come along for the ride. Another look at osteomalacia, then we will be on our way . . . painfully . . . slowly. If you suffer from chronic pain, this chapter may alter the course of your life.

More on osteomalacia

One study showed that 93% of persons 10 to 65 years of age who were admitted to a hospital emergency department with muscle aches and bone pain and who had a wide variety of diagnoses, including fibromyalgia, chronic fatigue syndrome, and depression, were deficient in vitamin D. **~Holick, 2007**

*Hypovitaminosis D myopathy is a prominent symptom of vitamin D deficiency, and **severely** impaired muscle function may be present **before** biochemical signs of bone disease develop.* **~Glerup et al., 2000, emphasis added**

While a low vitamin D state can lead to both osteomalacia and osteoporosis, it just so happens that, of the two, only osteomalacia is painful (Holick, 2008), that is until you fracture a leg or break a hip—then look out! ***Then*** osteoporosis is painful, very painful! Unfortunately, the only definitive way to determine the presence of osteomalacia vs. osteoporosis is by having a bone biopsy. (**"Ouch!"**— actually "Ouch." It hurts only a little.) However, there is another way to diagnose osteomalacia, a simple test offering a high degree of accuracy. Dr. Holick will tell you how: *"Osteomalacia can often be diagnosed by* using moderate force to press the sternum or anterior tibia, which can elicit bone pain." (Holick, 2007) This test is a great screening tool. If positive, it will suggest that your pain may be due to vitamin D deficiency and that you are, as a consequence, suffering from osteomalacia. Let's move on. I think I have covered osteomalacia sufficiently enough, at least for now.

Back pain

> Vitamin D insufficiency is common; repletion of vitamin D to normal levels in patients who have chronic low back pain or have had failed back surgery may improve quality of life or, in some cases, result in **complete** resolution of symptoms.   ~**Schwalfenberg, 2009, emphasis added**

> Among these patients, severe musculoskeletal pain involving the low back, neck, shoulders, hips, and legs was refractory to opioid [narcotic] analgesic and nonsteroidal anti-inflammatory medications [NSAIDs] but resolved following vitamin D repletion.   ~**Turner et al., 2008**

If you doubt whether a chronic low vitamin D state could be a prevalent cause of severe back pain, I may be able to straighten you out. I have several case reports laid out before me; I am bent over ("Ouch!") looking at them now—and all are from reputable sources, available free online for all to read. They speak of significant to complete resolution of low back pain, in both young and elderly patients, when low vitamin D levels are identified and corrected. The lesson here: Hypovitaminosis D can lead to devastating, narcotic-seeking, narcotic-dependent back pain. The never-getting-better kind of life-dominating and life-destroying back pain, and the back pain that vanished (or was significantly reduced) once a low vitamin D level was corrected—often within a matter of weeks! These case reports include histories of failed back surgeries followed by successful surgeries once vitamin D repletion and bone healing were achieved. Go online; read these papers for yourself. Here, I will give you a brief summary of 7 cases that demonstrate, with respect to chronic back pain, that remarkable results can be achieved with vitamin D repletion.

Case #1: Back pain, age 78, long-term duration, initial vitamin level of 2.2 ng/ml, complete resolution occurred within 4 weeks after vitamin D status normalized to 52 ng/ml. (Ghose, 2004a)

Case #2: Back pain, age 86, of three months duration and associated with a history of lumbar compression fractures. Vitamin D level was increased from ≤5 ng/ml to 36 ng/ml with pain resolution occurring following 3 weeks of treatment. (Ghose, 2004b)

Case #3: Back pain, age 47, long-term duration, with return of back pain 6 months after disc surgery. Initial vitamin D level was estimated at 28 ng/ml. Complete resolution occurred in 4 weeks after vitamin D level was increased to 48 ng/ml. Pain returned after the patient stopped taking vitamin D and again resolved after vitamin D supplementation was resumed. (Schwalfenberg, 2009)

Case #4: Back pain, age 44, back spasms allowed only limited activity. Complete resolution of back pain and spasms occurred following treatment of 5,000 IU/day of vitamin D to raise her vitamin D level from 19.6 ng/ml to 68.4 ng/ml. (Schwalfenberg, 2009)

Case #5: Back pain, age 30, chronic and disabling. Symptoms increased after a pregnancy but resolved completely after her vitamin D level was raised from 7.2 ng/ml to 28.8 ng/ml. (Schwalfenberg, 2009)

Case #6: Back pain, age 63, with a history of 4 back operations (**"Ouch!"**). He received the diagnosis "failed back surgery" and his self-esteem plummeted (well, it probably did). He was on long-term disability and attended a pain management clinic. He was a total mess! *"His symptoms completely resolved after six weeks on 4,000*

IU of vitamin D [per day] after years of having pain." His initial vitamin D level was 8 ng/ml. After treatment, his level rose to 34.8 ng/ml. (Schwalfenberg, 2009)

Case #7: Back pain, age 46. Chronic back pain continued following a lumbar fusion. This patient was screwed! A reoperation was required at 6 weeks post op. Screws that had been used the initial surgery were found to be loose. *"The bone was noted to be softer than normal and the fusion was not sound."* His initial vitamin D level was <4.8 ng/ml. Following treatment to raise his vitamin D level to 50 ng/ml, his symptoms were *"much improved."* (Plehwe and Carey, 2002)

In the above case reports, I took the liberty to convert the nmol/L, as found in the references, to ng/ml. Since ng/ml is the value that you will most likely see on a laboratory report, this conversion should help you better relate to the above case reports. I will also perform this conversion in the other case reports I have included in this chapter.

The examples above illustrate what *may* be possible if hypovitaminosis D is identified and effectively treated in those who present with chronic back pain. Of course, not every case will respond as in the examples above, but who knows how many will? One cannot simply dismiss the above case reports as an aberration—particularly in context with the study I am about to relate.

In this study, 360 chronic back pain patients were clinically evaluated. **83%** were found to have low vitamin D levels ranging from <4 ng/ml to 8.96 ng/ml. After an initial evaluation, all study participants were given 5,000 to 10,000 IU/d of vitamin D. The result: *"341 patients (95%) reported disappearance of low back pain after vitamin D therapy."* (Al Faraj and Al Mutairi, 2003) The physicians conducting this study call their results *"a remarkable clinical and biochemical response to oral therapy with vitamin D."* I believe they are, indeed, correct.

The above study took place in sunny Saudi Arabia, where low levels of vitamin D are commonplace due to cultural practices, and the fact that no one wants to be fried like an egg (or burnt to a crisp) in the desert sun! It goes without saying that back pain sufferers do not usually live a lifestyle that gets them involved in outdoor, daytime activities. They live their lives on the couch. They cherish the remote! They have watched every episode of *Gilligan's Island,* god knows how many times! And, like the rest of us, they probably do not get enough vitamin D in their diet to make up for the lack of vitamin D they would normally be receiving from regular sunlight exposure—who walking (or sitting) among us can eat 5 to 10 cans of tuna per day? The authors of this study close by saying: ***"Screening for vitamin D deficiency should be performed for all patients with chronic low back pain."*** (Emphasis added) Have you been screened? Do you live a life in the shadows?

It is important to note that the patients in Saudi Arabia had *chronic* back pain from—guess what?—osteomalacia! The authors of the study write: *"Chronic low back pain has been documented well as a presenting symptom of osteomalacia."* So, don't tell me that osteomalacia is "rare"! It can be found, in varying degrees, in perhaps millions of people lying on the couch and in those who are painfully walking among us—not just chronic back pain patients but fibromyalgia patients as well! It is simply not identified for what it is. But it will be if I have anything to say about it!

More aches and pains

> Myopathy, due to chronic vitamin D deficiency, probably contributes to immobility and ill health in a significant number of patients in the northern United States. ***~Prabhala et al., 2000***

In a paper by Prabhala et al, which can be found in the *Archives of Internal Medicine* (a highly respected medical journal that sometimes gathers dust), they report on 5 cases involving severe pain and muscle weakness. All 5 patients were basically wheelchair-bound. As before, I will briefly summarize each case as follows:

Case #1: Age 37, aches and pains with increasing weakness, confined to a wheelchair. She had peripheral neuropathy due to type 1 diabetes. Her initial vitamin D level was 4.8 ng/ml. After 6 weeks of 50,000 IU/wk of D2, her vitamin D level was 55.6 ng/ml and *"she lost her aches and pains, regained her strength, became mobile in 3 to 4 weeks, and is now able to walk and climb stairs."*

Case #2: Age 71, history of severe leg pain, muscle weakness, and difficulty walking. Included in his diagnosis was diabetic neuropathy. After treatment that brought his vitamin D level from 11.2 ng/ml to 74.8 ng/ml, *"his weakness and bone pains resolved within 6 weeks. He currently walks 2 to 3 blocks on his own without support."* He tells everyone around him, *"Please, I beg of you, do not slap sunscreen on the youngins!"*

Case #3: Age 77, confined to a wheelchair, with a vitamin D level of 4.8 ng/ml. *"She was given oral ergocalciferol [D₂] (50,000 IU/wk), with a dramatic improvement in her aches and pains. There was improved mobility, decreased weakness, and ability to forsake the wheelchair in 6 weeks."* The wheelchair was put up for sale on eBay.

Case #4: Age 67, with *"severe, painful proximal myopathy at the hip girdle."* This unfortunate lady has a life complicated by metastatic cancer. After being treated with 50,000 IU/wk of D₂, her vitamin D level went from 4.8 ng/ml to 16.8 ng/ml. *"Her pain and weakness improved significantly in 8 weeks."*

Case #5: Age 46. *"She was referred for severe pain all over her body"* and was described as *"frail."* She purchased a used wheelchair online (eBay, I think it was) and used it to get around. She reported *"each movement was painful."* She was a _total_ disaster! Her baseline level of vitamin D was 12.8 ng/ml. She was given a 50,000 IU D₂ injection and *"four weeks after the dose of* *vitamin D, her weakness had improved, and she was able to walk with support."*

Someone was clearly paying attention here! (And doing the right thing.) Impressively, in the above examples, low vitamin D levels were found in people you would think could *never* improve. There are hundreds, if not thousands, of individuals suffering in similar fashion in every major city and throughout the realm. Will they get the help they need? No. Well, maybe. But probably not. But maybe.

Back to basics

While there is no substitute for correcting structural abnormalities with surgery and improving function with physical therapy, if inflammation is involved—and it will be!—there is also <u>no</u> substitute for decisively dealing with inflammation. Chronic back pain, sustained by a state of chronic inflammation, is one major health problem here in America. And back pain is not always caused by physical trauma or pathological alteration. The gods may be exceptionally angry, and chronic inflammation is probably playing a subtle role. Sometimes, inflammation can be reduced by a walking program. Losing weight can often be helpful in relieving chronic back pain, and it is helpful in this regard for several reasons. But other times you can just forget it! <u>Nothing</u> seems to help! And, all too often, narcotics come along, take over a life . . . and ruin it. However, I can share with you a treatment option for back pain that has shown real promise, as follows:

An omega-3 protocol

It is possible to reduce back pain by including more omega-3 fatty acids (found abundantly in fish oils) in your diet. The omega-3 fatty acids are highly anti-inflammatory. And, knowing you, your intake of the omega-3s is nothing to brag about. You may find help and motivation by reading the following:

—**Maroon JC, Bost RW** 2006 w-3 Fatty Acids (Fish Oil) as an Anti-inflammatory: An Alternative to Nonsteroidal Anti-inflammatory Drugs for Discogenic Pain. Surgical Neurology 65:326–331

For more on this topic, I invite you to read the following:

—**Maroon JC Bost, JW, Maroon A** 2010 Natural Anti-inflammatory Agents for Pain Relief. Surg Neurol Int 1:80 doi:10.4103/2152-7806.73804

—**Ko GD, Nowacki NB, Arseneau L, Eitel M, Hum A** 2010 Omega-3 Fatty Acids for Neuropathic Pain *Case Series*. Clin J Pain; February; 26(2):168–172

More case reports to share, 5 in all

The following paper on vitamin D deficiency and pain is not available free at this point in time. Your physician or a medical librarian can order it for you. It relates the experiences of 5 individuals who were admitted to a nursing home. I will summarize as follows:

Case #1: Age 86, weak and malnourished. She was admitted to the nursing home with severe lower extremity pain. Her vitamin D level was 5 ng/ml. Twenty some days later, and following restorative nutrition along with vitamin D replacement of 700 IU/day, her *"pain had subsided completely."* Following treatment, her vitamin D level rose to 35 ng/ml.

Case #2: Age 68 (like this is old!). This gentleman was confined at home a number of years to a *"dark and dingy bedroom"* and was too weak to walk. He would cry out in pain from time to time and avoided all physical activity. Pain limited his mobility and even occurred with a light touch to the skin. His vitamin D level was found to be at 12.8 ng/ml. After one week following an initial 50,000 IU of vitamin D and 400 IU/day, *"his pain vanished."*

Case #3: Age 94 (I think we're talkin' old, now). This lady had recently suffered a broken hip and was admitted to the nursing home for continuing care. One complaint was severe lower leg pain. Her vitamin D level was a mere 3.2 ng/ml (extremely low). She received both vitamin D and calcium supplementation and within 5 days reported improvement, even with only a minor increase of her vitamin D level to 4.4 ng/ml. Her need of pain medication was greatly reduced.

Case #4: Age 85 and counting. She was admitted to the nursing home following a 3 month stay in the hospital to undergo treatment for a lung infection. She suffered *"intense"* pain in both legs and feet. Each leg was tender to the touch. She did not like her feet anymore, for they were not happy feet. Her vitamin D level was 4.1 ng/ml. Following a 50,000 IU dose of oral vitamin D, she reported noticeable improvement in her level of pain.

Case #5: Age 24 (I think we're talkin' young). This is a sad case. It will rip your heart out. This young lady suffered an infection involving her spinal nerves that left her quadriplegic and in a state of reduced consciousness. She needed a tracheostomy for breathing and a tube for feeding. She was on Phenobarbital, a drug known to lower vitamin D levels, to control her seizures. Even though she could not move, she could still feel pain. She was tested for hypovitaminosis D. Her vitamin level was 8 ng/ml. Within 1 week following treatment, her pain resolved. Her repeat vitamin D level was 24.8 ng/ml. Two months later, her pain returned. Her vitamin D level had dropped to 12 ng/ml. Again, after treatment, her pain was relieved.

Reference cited:

—**Gloth III FM, Lindsay JM, Zelesnick LB, Greenough III WB** 1991 Can Vitamin D Produce an Unusual Pain Syndrome? Arch Intern Med; August; 151:1662–1664

The authors of this study make the following recommendation:

At this juncture, it seems prudent to consider an assessment of vitamin D status before initiating pain control measures, such as narcotics and antidepressants. This information is particularly important for the homebound elderly or for those confined to nursing homes.

I couldn't agree more. The elderly and the institutionalized are sitting ducks when it comes to vitamin D deficiency, and sometimes with devastating consequences. This is often a neglected population, and the suffering can be intense. Later in life, it could happen to you.

Chapter 17
Obesity

Nearly one third of all U.S. adults are categorized as obese. ~**Parikh et al., 2004**

Obesity is often associated with vitamin D deficiency. It is now recognized that, whether vitamin D is ingested or obtained from exposure to sunlight, it is efficiently deposited in the large body fat stores and is not bioavailable. This is probably the reason that obese persons are chronically vitamin D deficient. ~**Holick, 2004**

B ecause of the *weight* and significance of this issue—obesity—you might think that this would be a *big*, perhaps *enormous,* chapter, *stuffed full* of facts and *figures* that serve to give the reader a *broad* understanding of the subject. (Sorry, I just couldn't resist throwing in a few puns.) But, in an effort to move things along, I will comment only *a little* on this issue. One *small* paragraph should be all that it takes to obtain an *adequate* understanding of the relationship between obesity and vitamin D. This is serious business! A *big* deal! Pay attention! I'll be *brief.*

If you are truly obese—not the "little overweight" business that some people call "obesity"—vitamin D adequacy is very hard to achieve. Diet is simply not enough. Your skin is a little thicker than the skin of those of lesser abundance, impeding the penetration of UVB radiation to a relevant degree (Cantor, 2008). Any vitamin D that is produced awaits a predictable fate. Fat cells, it seems, want nothing more than to store vitamin D for a rainy day (Holick, 2002; Holick, 2004), but this will make it *largely* unavailable for use by other cells and other cellular processes. In addition, the obese patient is less likely to go outdoors, less likely to expose skin to any relevant degree, and less likely to participate in outdoor, sun-exposure activities. So Plan B is just about it! And, although you are obese, you do seem to squeak by. There is at least some vitamin D in your diet that keeps you going and going and going (slowly), but not enough to keep you out of trouble in the long run with respect to vitamin D. Vitamin D deficiency in obesity is no piece of cake, no picnic! It is very serious business and a *bigger* problem than one can imagine. **You** are the <u>*ultimate*</u> indoor person! Even when you are outside, you are inside! **You** are hidden from view by layers of— well, you know! And you *will* pay a price. **You**, perhaps more than anyone walking slowly among us, need vitamin D to be in adequate supply. **You** need Plan B, and you need it done right—period!

Bottom line: Get tested! Get treated! Get retested! Repeat the cycle—particularly if you are obese. Maintain an adequate vitamin D level . . . throughout life. Don't let your guard down! Achieve and maintain a respectable vitamin D level. Are we clear? Are we?

The skinny on obesity

If you would like to learn what is behind the obesity epidemic in our society, and what to do about it, watch the following video series. It may be the most important series of videos you can watch, period! It is produced by the University of California, so it can probably be trusted. You just <u>have</u> to watch this series. I insist! You can search YouTube for each individual video by name. Or, better yet, go to the first web address listed below and watch the entire series, episode by episode, right from the official website.

—**The Skinny on Obesity (EP. 1): An Epidemic for Every Body**
www.uctv.tv/skinny-on-obesity/

—**The Skinny on Obesity (EP. 2): Sickeningly Sweet**

Problems after gastric bypass, a case report

Let's hope you *never* find yourself in this kind of trouble. This is the story of a most unfortunate lady, age 64. She had undergone gastric bypass at age 58 and had lost 100 pounds yet remained severely obese. She presented with diffuse muscle and bone pain, pain she had experienced for several years and varied in intensity from day to day. The pain was especially pronounced in her rib cage. All of this was very concerning because she had breast cancer one year after her gastric bypass and soon thereafter underwent a modified radical mastectomy. The worry now was that her pain was from metastatic cancer to the bone. *"A bone scan, obtained because of concern about metastatic malignancy, revealed areas of increased activity in the right hip, the right inferior pubic ramus, and multiple left ribs, interpreted as consistent with metastases."* Also worrisome was an elevated alkaline phosphatase of 231 (normal range is 39–117), an elevation that can occur with a serious, active disease process involving the bone. Things would change for this lady and fears would subside. Appropriate labs were drawn. As a result, her vitamin D level was found to be *"undetectable"* and her PTH level was significantly elevated, presumably in response. She was started on high-dose vitamin D along with calcium supplementation. After three months of treatment her rib pain resolved and remained resolved when reevaluated four months later.

The resolution of her rib pain occurred even though her vitamin D status still remained low at 15 ng/ml.

Comment: Gastric bypass is a "red flag" when it comes to an individual's vitamin D status. This procedure purposefully limits the intake and absorption of food and nutrients in order to promote weight loss. Accordingly, the amount of vitamin D absorbed from food sources is greatly decreased following gastric bypass. This is, undoubtedly, the reason why her vitamin D status became so severely compromised. Two things in particular make this case noteworthy. First, she had a fairly rapid turnaround in her symptoms following vitamin D replacement. And, second, this case of vitamin D deficiency masqueraded as metastatic bone cancer. This individual still has health challenges to face but has been relieved of one very serious concern, that of bone cancer. Bone cancer is an extremely serious matter. But then, so is hypovitaminosis D. The reference below presents three similar case reports of vitamin D deficiency masquerading as metastatic cancer.

—**Khokhar JS, Brett AS, Desai A** 2009 Vitamin D Deficiency Masquerading as Metastatic Cancer: A Case Series. The American Journal of the Medical Sciences; April; 337(4):245–247

A surprising relationship

Surprisingly, lack of sleep can lead to weight gain. Studies confirm that those who receive inadequate sleep (for whatever reason), gain more weight than those who receive an adequate amount of sleep. Does less sleep equal more time for eating? (There is always time for more eating.) No, this is not the answer. Sleep loss alters the hormones that regulate our perception of hunger and satiety. Basically, when you are sleep deprived, you are "told" by certain hormones, and with more intensity, that you are starving to death (when it is obvious that you are not—just look at you!). Due to a dysfunctional hormonal drive, you eat more than you should. Furthermore, the hormonal imbalance that occurs with sleep loss increases insulin resistance in skeletal muscle. As a result, the message goes out that you need more fuel (when you really don't—you have plenty of fuel on board). In this situation, more insulin is released in order to help drive glucose into muscle; unfortunately, insulin also acts to drive excess calories into storage as fat. Sleep loss is nothing to dismiss as inconsequential. It adds to the epidemic of obesity we find ourselves in. Yes, the epidemic that is destroying the lives of so many. (I will miss them.) This story is told in the following papers.

—*Web*MD 2010 Sleep and Weight Gain: Will Better Sleep Help You Avoid Extra Pounds?
www.webmd.com/sleep-disorders/excessive-sleepiness-10/lack-of-sleep-weight-gain

—Patel SR, Malhotra A, White DP, Gottlieb DJ, Hu FB 2006 Association between Sleep and Weight Gain. Am J Epidemiol; November 15; 164(10):947–954

—Taheri S, Lin L, Austin D, Young T, Mignot E 2004 Short Sleep Duration Is Associated with Reduced Leptin, Elevated Ghrelin, and Increased Body Mass Index. PLoS Medicine; December; 1(3):210–217

Chapter 18
Spare the children

Regular and sensible sun exposure during the months of the year when vitamin D production is promoted is still the most physiologic way to prevent vitamin D deficiency in infants and children.   ~**Holick, 2006**

Because there is little, if any, vitamin D in human milk, infants, especially infants of women of color, are at high risk of developing vitamin D deficiency and rickets if they are not given a vitamin D supplement. ~**Holick, 2004**

Hollis et al. reported that giving lactating females 4,000 IU vitamin D3 daily provides adequate vitamin D in breast milk to satisfy the infant's requirement.   ~**Holick, 2006**

For a lactating mother, it is essential that sustained circulating vitamin D be maintained.

We understand more fully now that this deficiency [hypovitaminosis D associated with breastfeeding] is not caused by something inherently wrong or missing in mother's milk but rather by inadequate maternal dietary vitamin D intake and the resultant low concentrations in the mother's milk.   ~**Wagner et al., 2008, emphasis added**

This chapter will be by far the most important chapter in the entire book. What *ever* could be more important than preventing disease in children and preventing their tragic loss? (I knew you couldn't think of a thing.) Vitamin D can do this, if supplies are adequate. But we as a society are raising yet another generation of indoor people, shielding them from sunlight in a variety of ways and failing to compensate with adequate vitamin D supplementation. There *will* be a price to pay. And sometimes the price is paid at a tender young age.   Juvenile-onset diabetes is a case in point. It is a very serious disease, well worth preventing. We'll start the conversation here.

Type I Diabetes

Vitamin D deficiency in utero and during the first year of life has also been linked to increased risk of type 1 diabetes. **~Holick, 2006**

Juvenile-onset diabetes, now called type 1 diabetes, occurs when the insulin-producing cells of the pancreas are destroyed by an individual's own immune system. A life is forever changed. Perhaps a bacterial insult sets the stage, and the cells of the pancreas become the unintended victim. Unfortunately, this disease is not all that rare. There are thousands upon thousands of our kids with type 1 diabetes, millions worldwide! Alarmingly, there are approximately **15,000 new cases diagnosed <u>each year</u> in the United States alone!** And, yes, I do know how serious this disease is. One of my high school classmates gradually went blind, had sequential foot followed by sequential leg amputations, and eventually died at a relatively young age—all because of this dreadful disease. The image of my former classmate, sitting in a wheel chair, blind and without legs, is certainly not a pleasant one. And there is a good chance that none of this should have occurred! **Pay close attention to what follows.**

We now know that type 1 diabetes can, *in great measure*, be prevented by adequate vitamin D supplementation during infancy. ***"Children in Finland in the 1960s who received the recommended 2,000 IU of vitamin D/day at least during the first year of life and followed for the next 31 years demonstrated a reduced risk of developing type 1 diabetes by <u>80%</u>."*** (Holick, 2006, emphasis added) **80%!** *Impressive!* Yet we remain of the belief that the recommended 200, 400, even 600 IU of vitamin D per day is all that is needed by infant and child. We seldom adjust recommendations or degree of supplementation by factoring in winter, latitude, diet, poverty, race, or the use of sunscreen.

And just like that, we condemn many to a life of vitamin D deficiency and increased risk of some very serious and unpleasant diseases. It is that easy. And even with the impressive care medicine has to offer the type 1 diabetic today, kids still die from this disease. Not necessarily when they are still young (although it does happen), but particularly as they get older. Alarmingly, the death rate is *seven times* the death rate of those who do not have the disease. And *"women with type 1 diabetes are 13 times more likely to die [prematurely from disease] than women who did not have diabetes."* (source: American Diabetes Association, 2010, emphasis added) These disturbing statistics speak to the need to do whatever it takes to prevent this evil from occurring. But are we, as parents, and are we as a society, doing whatever it takes? (You can answer the question if you want to.)

I highlight type 1 diabetes here because it is such a glaring example of the impact vitamin D deficiency has on our children. But there are other risks and other problems that lie in wait, all related to vitamin D deficiency. As we continue, we will take a look at how a chronic lack of vitamin D can complicate and challenge the lives of the innocent. Some of what follows will be a review. We'll start before the child is born. And you'll get to meet Charlie.

Gestation-related risks

At no time in human nutrition is it more critical to ensure nutrient intake than during the state of pregnancy.

The current recommended dietary requirement for vitamin D intake during pregnancy and lactation is based on little, if any, scientific evidence, and as a result is clinically irrelevant with respect to maintaining nutritional vitamin D status during these demanding human conditions. Current research has shown that the actual dietary requirement during pregnancy and lactation may actually be as high as 6,000 IU/d. ~**Hollis, 2007**

Adequate vitamin D intake is essential for maternal and fetal health during pregnancy, and epidemiological data indicate that many pregnant *women have sub-optimal vitamin D levels. Notably, vitamin D deficiency correlates with **preeclampsia, gestational diabetes mellitus, and bacterial vaginosis, and an increased risk of C-section delivery.** Recent work emphasizes the importance of nonclassical roles of vitamin D in pregnancy and the placenta. The placenta produces and responds to vitamin D where vitamin D functions as a modulator of implantation, cytokine production and the **immune response to infection.*** ~Shin et al., 2010, **emphasis added**

We have, in the past, received some very poor advice with respect to vitamin D during pregnancy and lactation, advice with absolutely no scientific backing (they just guessed at it—see Hollis and Wagner, 2006a). Fortunately, things are changing, but progress is slow and even the best recommendation can simply be ignored, one mom at a time.

Not only does vitamin D protect the fetus from game-changing infectious disease, vitamin D promotes normal fetal development. Charlie, whom we haven't seen just yet, will need vitamin D in adequate supply from "Mom" or his health, quality of development, even his survival, could be at risk. Many die before birth simply due to vitamin D deficiency in the mother-to-be. This is so true. This is so sad. But, luckily for Charlie, the little guy of our story, vitamin D levels in "Mom," although nothing to brag about, were somehow sufficient—***He made it out alive!*** However, during gestation, subtle and not so subtle problems certainly could have developed.

Charlie has just been born (**Ouch!**). He's a little unsightly (and slippery) at the moment, but this will last for only a few minutes, and Charlie will be transformed into perhaps the most beautiful thing his parents have ever seen (aside from those funny little depressions on his head called craniotabes—perhaps the first sign that Charlie is vitamin D deficient right from the start). (see Yorifuju et al., 2008)

Yes, things went pretty well for Charlie, overall. But bad things could have happened to him if "Mom" had been very low in vitamin D during his gestation, like millions of pregnant women throughout the world. So what bad things could have happened to Charlie, the beautiful little baby boy of our story?

Gestational issues related to vitamin D deficiency can be summarized as follows:

- **Preeclampsia.** This is a serious condition that kills the unborn and makes people very sad. This disease is characterized by high blood pressure in the mother-to-be, a situation that can lead to uterine bleeding and premature separation of the placenta from the uterine wall. The condition is resolved with premature delivery of the placenta along with delivery of the fetus. And, should the fetus be viable following this untimely turn of events, this situation results in the challenge of prematurity. Vitamin D is not the whole story here but is at least part of the story. One study demonstrated a *"27% reduction in the risk of preeclampsia in women receiving 400-600 IU/day of vitamin D from supplements at midpregnancy compared to women not reporting supplementation."* (Dror and Allen, 2010) By the way, moms die from this condition, too.

- **Bacterial vaginosis.** We have discussed this before in *Chapter 11.* Vitamin D protects against infections that harm the fetus. Mom can better protect her unborn child if she is creating defensive antimicrobials like cathelicidin, thereby preventing infectious organisms from reaching and colonizing the placenta and compromising the health and threatening the life of the fetus.

- **Gestational diabetes.** This problem, too, complicates the lives of both mother and fetus. Both have an increased risk of developing type 2 diabetes later in life, with an increased risk of obesity awaiting the one yet to be born (Grundmann and von Versen-Höynk, 2011). Stillbirths and congenital defects can occur in extreme cases. In addition, gestational diabetes leads to large birth weight (**Ouch!**). (see Kjos and Buchanan, 1999) One study relates a low vitamin D level in "Mom" with a 2.7-fold increase in gestational diabetes (Grundmann and von Versen-Höynk, 2011).

- **Developmental disorders.** These are a range of problems that have their beginnings in the womb, associated with vitamin D deficiency. They include low birth weight, improper skeletal development with an increased risk of osteoporosis later in life (Grundmann and von Versen-Höynk, 2011), and delayed motor development (Munns et al., 2006). And, as we have previously discussed, vitamin D deficiency can lay the foundation for conditions such as autism and schizophrenia.

That's enough! I'm depressed. But Charlie's not depressing, he's so damn cute! And even though he escaped most if not all of the gestational problems that could have occurred before his day of birth, he is still at risk of some very bad things should he remain vitamin D deficient. And I, like you, are deeply worried over Charlie.

After birth and beyond

Although Charlie seems to be "okay" for the moment, he *was* born vitamin D deficient. This is concerning. And his cuteness will not come to his aid at all in this respect. Furthermore, what's on tap (breast milk) will not help him to any great degree here either. I don't see Charlie's mom getting outside very much, not with a new-born baby to take care of and all. And her physician is old school and not really into vitamin D, and he may not even know that it takes up to **2,000 to 6,400 IUs** of vitamin D, per day, in "Mom" for a satisfactory amount of vitamin D to show up her breast milk (Hollis and Wagner, 2004; Wagner et al., 2008). So, as cute as he is, Charlie will be sick a lot—including ear infections and diseases that involve the prodigious production of snot—perhaps related to ongoing vitamin D deficiency. He looks kinda sickly, don't you think?

There are a few things that have contributed to Charlie's vitamin D deficiency that I didn't mention. He was conceived in August, a time when vitamin D levels in "Mom" should be the highest, and he was born in May, a time when vitamin D levels in "Mom" are typically quite low. Winter was not particularly kind to Charlie, and much of his gestation occurred when vitamin D levels are typically low in mothers-to-be. There's something else: Charlie's mother is, at baseline, quite overweight—a situation that typically impairs the conversion of sunlight into vitamin D and acts to deny both mother and fetus of vitamin D sufficiency. It really is that simple. But, luckily for both Mom and Charlie, it will soon be summer, a season of atonement with respect to low vitamin D. (But only if we can get them outdoors and into the sunshine.) If the "Charlie and Mom duo" do things right, I see a sizable amount of vitamin D coming their way. However, I do not expect to see any show up in Mom's breast milk unless she is taking vitamin D supplements in a daily dose sufficient to compensate for her weight, with enough left over to wind its way into her milk supply. So Charlie is bound to remain vitamin D deficient until next summer when he can run around in his diaper in the sunshine (as fast as his wobbly little legs will carry him). Oh, how I wish Charlie were getting more vitamin D . . . from somewhere! A vitamin D supplement would certainly be nice and a wise course of action. Let's hope Charlie's mom is giving him some kind of supplement to tide him over until next summer; some is better than none.

Sadly, many, many infants and young children, even in the most developed nation on the planet, get little if any vitamin D by supplementation, nor do they receive anywhere near an adequate amount of vitamin D per sunshine exposure. So, like little Charlie, many are at risk of problems they could certainly live without. Some, like Charlie's future classmate Jimmy, will come down with type 1 diabetes. And Billie over there will come down with Crohn's. Suzie probably won't come down with MS, but her best friend Sarah will. How sad.

So, what are the health risks that our children face, problems strongly associated hypovitaminosis D? I will list a few, taken, in part, from a nice little paper written by Munns et al.

- Rickets, abnormal skeletal development, increased risk of fractures. And, yes, osteomalacia. Apparently this disease is not just limited to adults. Recall, osteomalacia causes muscle aches and pains.

- Delayed tooth eruption, and abnormal development of tooth enamel (leading to tooth decay and loss).

- Increased risk of infectious diseases, including diseases involving snot (in prodigious amounts).

- Increased risk of type 1 diabetes.

- Increased risk of asthma.

- Increased risk of Crohn's disease (Pappa et al., 2006; Sentongo et al., 2002).

Hypovitaminosis D during gestation, infancy, and childhood is a risk factor for problems that show up, unexpectedly, later in life. These include:

- Hypertension

- Cardiovascular disease

- Type 2 diabetes

- Obesity

- Cancer

- Multiple sclerosis

That's enough. I'm in overload! There are so many medical conditions related to vitamin D deficiency that it is crazy! So, how crazy is it to want people, no matter their age—even the unborn!—to be sufficient in vitamin D? And I haven't even mentioned childhood cancer.

> Children exposed to the most sunlight had a **40% reduced risk** of developing non-Hodgkin lymphoma. (Holick, 2006, emphasis added)

Although there is only a little information available on the relationship between vitamin D deficiency and childhood cancer, the above quotation suggests that such a relationship does indeed exist. But let's not wait for all the data to be in before we act. Many are the reasons to provide our precious little children with the gift of vitamin D sufficiency . . . even before they are born. Cancer should probably be included on the list.

Let's end our discussion with this . . .

> Why should anyone be concerned about vitamin D deficiency during pregnancy? After all, the skeletal problems encountered appear to be corrected simply by vitamin D supplementation after delivery. The answer is simple: the function of vitamin D is now known to extend well beyond skeletal integrity, and thus it would be a tragedy to ignore this information. (Hollis and Wagner, 2006b)

Diabetes was once rare, once upon a time

And I quote:

> At the start of the 20th century, child diabetes was rare and rapidly fatal. By its end, some 3–4 children per 1,000 in Western countries would require insulin treatment by age 20 years, and a steady rise in incidence had been reported from many other parts of the world.
>
> Diabetes itself was an uncommon diagnosis in the 19th century. (Gale, 2002)

It's true, in the past both type 1 and type 2 diabetes were seen here and there, but not regularly, and they were nowhere near as prevalent as they are today—then the 21st century came along! Now even type 2 diabetes, previously called adult-onset diabetes, is increasingly found in children!

> Although considered uncommon a few decades ago, type 2 diabetes in adolescents now represents one of the most rapidly growing forms of diabetes in the United States and perhaps worldwide. (Ponder et al., 2000)

So, why the change? I actually have a good idea. A low vitamin D status is certainly in there somewhere (you've heard of sunscreen, you've heard of winter, you've heard of TV and video games that keep kids indoors, you've heard of . . .). Another reason for this alarming rise in both type 1 and type 2 diabetes is the rise in obesity, stemming in part from our Western diet. The following papers will help you get up to speed on these issues:

—**Gale E** 2002 The Rise of Childhood Type 1 Diabetes in the 20th Century. Diabetes; December; 51:3353–3361

— **Ponder SW, Sulivan S, McBath G** 2000 Type 2 Diabetes Mellitus in Teens. Diabetes Spectrum 13(2):95

—**Palomer X, et al** 2007 Role of Vitamin D in the Pathogenesis of Type 2 Diabetes Mellitus. Diabetes, Obesity and Metabolism; 10:185–197

Chapter 19
Now look here!

Age-related Macular Degeneration (AMD), a progressive degenerative condition of the retina, is the leading cause of legal blindness among older Americans. In the United States, 7 million individuals older than 40 years are diagnosed with early AMD and 1.7 million have advanced stages.

Consistent users of vitamin D-containing supplements in a subgroup of people consuming less than one serving of milk daily had decreased prevalent early AMD.

We speculate that vitamin D may reduce the risk of AMD by its anti-inflammatory properties. **~Parekh et al., 2007**

I had a tough time deciding just where in the book I should place this chapter. So, for no particular reason, you'll find it right here. Since there is not a lot of information currently available on the topic of vitamin D and vision health, this chapter will be over in the blink of an eye! Let's *see*, now where do we begin?

The vitamin that you normally think of when it comes to vision is, of course, vitamin A. But don't underestimate the power of vitamin D! It seems that this vitamin, or as I like to remind folks, this hormone, plays a role in the health of the eye (or two). While we still can, I think we should take a look at macular degeneration, a major cause of blindness in adults age 50 and older.

Macular degeneration is a degenerative condition that affects the retina, the light-sensitive portion of the eye, and progressively restricts an individual's visual field. Some who are seriously affected by this condition can only listen to *Gilligan's Island* reruns and can only remember how beautiful Ginger really was (and still is).

As stated in the quotations at the beginning of this chapter, macular degeneration affects millions of individuals in the United States. My guess is, as a class, they are indoor people and have been deficient in vitamin D much of their lives. Even though there is not a lot of research available on this topic, paying attention to vitamin D and personally achieving a respectable level of this essential hormone—a measure that may improve the health of the eye—just makes sense. Vitamin D helps every other bodily system in many ways, why would it not be beneficial to the eye?

The authors cited at the beginning of the chapter, Parekh et al, have offered a couple of reasons why vitamin D may be helpful in preventing the leading cause of blindness, the disease we call macular degeneration. The ability of vitamin D to calm down inflammatory processes is one. The other, the ability of vitamin D to prevent abnormal patterns of growth. Both of which are implicated in the pathogenesis of this disease. Perhaps vitamin D deficiency increases the risk of eye damage known to occur from excessive sunlight exposure. In any event, I have a little advice to offer: Ask your eye care professional about the use of eye protection while out in the sunshine. He or she may not know the latest on vitamin D and the prevention of macular degeneration, but members of this profession sure know how to sell sunglasses! (Hint! You should probably be using UVB-blocking eye protection when you are in the sun for any extended period of time, as you are safely soaking up all of that vitamin D).

How to cheat on an eye exam

Remember, the first letter on the eye chart is almost always an **E**.

Chapter 20
Kidney failure

*Recently, it has become clear that 1,25(OH)$_2$D has potent immuno-modulatory and antiproliferative properties, suggesting a role for vitamin D in the pathophysiology of autoimmune disease, common cancers, hypertension, **renal inflammation**, and cardiovascular disease.*
~Zehnder et al., 2008, emphasis added

Increasing evidence has demonstrated a correlation between vitamin D-deficiency and progression of CKD [chronic kidney disease], and plasma vitamin D status is an independent inverse predictor of disease progression and death in patients with CKD. Thus <u>vitamin D-deficiency may in fact accelerate the progression of kidney disease</u>.

*Vitamin D and vitamin D analog therapy has shown **multiple beneficial effects** in both hemodialysis and non-dialysis CKD patients, leading to significant **survival advantage** for patients receiving therapy.* **~Li, 2010, emphasis added**

*Vitamin D has emerged as a vital compound in CKD with newly ascribed autocrine [cell supplying itself with a needed molecule] functions vastly different from its classical function in mineral homeostasis [normal balance]. **To ignore the significance of this vitamin and its potential impact on morbidity and mortality is no longer appropriate.*** **~Williams et al., 2009, emphasis added**

This chapter, too, could have been placed just about anywhere in the book, but I chose to place it here . . . for *some* reason. I just can't remember what it was—Oh, since kidney failure often shows up at the end of life, why not place this chapter near the end of the book? Good a reason as any! We'll go with that. Now let's save some kidneys.

Perhaps 2 or 3 decades ago (when my memory was better) it would have been a little crazy to suggest that vitamin D sufficiency could help protect the kidney from harm. But today it's a different story. Advances in research have revealed a role for vitamin D in protecting the kidney from disease and from failure. The decline and loss of kidney function is one very serious matter. You won't like kidney failure . . . but you won't be alone! Chronic kidney disease (CKD) affects, to some degree, approximately 1 out of every 10 Americans, 50 million individuals worldwide (Li, 2010).

Apart from direct and beneficial actions at the level of the kidney, vitamin D is also protective against medical conditions that can lead to kidney failure, conditions such as diabetes, lupus, cardiovascular disease, and hypertension. I mention diabetes first because *"Diabetes is by far the leading cause of CKD [chronic kidney disease]."* (Li, 2010) Other issues related to kidney failure, such as autoimmunity and vascular disease, may also be prevented or limited in severity by a life enriched by vitamin D.

But watch out for the subtle stuff! It has become evident that even low-grade systemic inflammation, such as is seen in obesity and living the insulin-resistant Western lifestyle (eating poorly with limited production or intake of vitamin D), can lead to slow, progressive loss of kidney function (Tang, et al., 2012; Kang et al., 2012). The kidneys are actually damaged by common, everyday low-grade inflammation . . . slowly . . . imperceptibly. Over time, kidney function begins to decline. Add an insult like diabetes, like hypertension, like progressive vascular disease, and you get to meet a nice new doctor. You may even progress to the point of requiring dialysis. You may like your new doctor, but you won't like dialysis.

In a previous discussion, we learned of the role the kidney plays in converting vitamin D into its active form, thereby providing a baseline level of the "active hormone" in the bloodstream for the benefit of other tissues and cells. Now it is apparent that this action also benefits the kidneys themselves. They, too, need vitamin D—converted into its active form and sufficiently available—in order to remain healthy and function as intended. Unfortunately, kidney disease can lead to a direct loss of vitamin D, leading to further compromise of an individual's vitamin D status. This clearly sounds like trouble.

One thing that occurs in chronic kidney disease is a slow, continual loss of protein in the urine. The kidneys can't help it, for they are diseased. Normally, vitamin D is bound to a certain protein as it moves from here to there in the bloodstream. Unfortunately, as protein is lost in the urine, from chronic kidney disease, so lost is vitamin D. Since the kidney itself needs vitamin D and vitamin D becomes increasingly less available (unless corrective measures are taken), kidney disease may be accelerated as a result (Li, 2010). A vicious cycle is created, with low vitamin D availability accelerating kidney disease, which in turn lowers vitamin D levels further, which in turn accelerates further kidney disease, which in turn . . . . The following tells this important story.

> Proteinuria [protein loss in the urine] . . . leads to loss of DBP-25OHD$_3$ [the vitamin D transport protein] in the urine and thus reduces the . . . uptake of 25OHD$_3$. Therefore it is not surprising that vitamin D-deficiency, particularly 1,25(OH)2D$_3$-deficiency, is commonly observed in patients with CKD even at the early stages of the disease because of impaired renal functions. Increasing evidence has demonstrated a correlation between vitamin D-deficiency of CKD, and plasma vitamin D status is an independent inverse predictor of disease progression and death in patients with CKD. Thus vitamin D-deficiency may in fact accelerate the progression of kidney disease. (Li, 2010)

Recall, our society is currently experiencing an epidemic of vitamin D deficiency. Add chronic disease of the kidney to the mix—a disease affecting 1 in 10 Americans—and we clearly have an epidemic within an epidemic! *"Patients with CKD have an exceptionally high rate of severe vitamin D deficiency that is further exacerbated by the reduced ability to convert 25-(OH)vitamin D into the active form."* (Williams et al., 2009) So is it any wonder that vitamin D deficiency is almost universal in those with chronic kidney disease? Something needs to be done! Thankfully, something is being done.

The patient undergoing treatment for chronic kidney disease today is probably no stranger to vitamin D supplementation. In this patient population the risk of accelerated cardiovascular disease, osteoporosis, and osteomalacia is clearly recognized and sometimes requires aggressive supplementation to forestall. *"Since vitamin D deficiency or insufficiency is highly prevalent, especially in patients with CKD, it should be managed aggressively even in early CKD."* (Tang, 2009) Accordingly, many are the treatment plans and strategies available to the physician. But keep in mind, in chronic kidney disease vitamin D replacement becomes a balancing act. Sometimes, vitamin D supplementation can raise blood calcium levels to inappropriately high levels, requiring a change in strategy, including dosage adjustment or the use of a vitamin D analog, one that limits the rise of calcium within the bloodstream (Tang, 2009). There are other problems, too, that may be encountered with vitamin D supplementation in the patient suffering from chronic kidney disease, making it a wise course of action for the kidney patient not to make adjustments in therapy without first consulting with his or her physician. It is also wise for the patient to report any negative effects experienced during the course of a vitamin D treatment regimen.

Today, while much focus is placed on vitamin D supplementation for those with chronic kidney disease, encouraging vitamin D sufficiency as a preventative measure for those who are at risk (that would be all of us) is generally lacking, allowing the epidemic of vitamin D deficiency to persist and claim victim after victim after victim after victim. And this epidemic clearly does have an impact on the health of the kidneys, in one individual at a time. Our society would have far less in the way of kidney disease if vitamin D deficiency were rare rather than the norm. This is clear. Yet, silently, the epidemic continues.

There is one more important issue that we should discuss before we leave this chapter behind. It concerns vitamin D and the kidney transplant patient. The kidney transplant patient is a "special-needs" patient when it comes to vitamin D. The use of anti-rejection meds generally dictates that one stay out of direct sunlight, due to an increased risk of skin cancer (Querings et al., 2006; Ewers et al., 2008). This precaution will undoubtedly lower vitamin D availability, placing this patient population at great risk of problems like osteomalacia and osteoporosis (Ewers et al., 2008; Boudville and Hodsman, 2006). So, similar to the kidney failure patient, the kidney transplant patient will need to be followed carefully with respect to his or her vitamin D status (Ewers et al., 2008).

Vitamin D analogues in CKD

It is common to see amodified form of vitamin D, called a vitamin D analog, prescribed for kidney failure patients. The goal here is to provide the patient with the benefits of the active form of vitamin D without the adverse effect of hypercalcemia (elevated blood calcium). Also, "recent studies demonstrate that vitamin D analogues have potent renoprotective effects." (Li, 2010) *Renoprotective* is another way of saying *kidney protective*. Paricalcitol (Zemplar), is the vitamin D analog most often prescribed. The following three papers are offered should one wish to learn more about vitamin D analogues.

—**Brown AJ** 2001 Therapeutic Uses of Vitamin D Analogues. American Journal of Kidney Diseases 38(5)(Suppl 5):S3–S19

—**Al-Badr W, Martin KJ** 2008 Vitamin D and Kidney Disease. Clin J Am Nephrol 3:1555–1560

—**Li YC** 2010 Renoprotective Effects of Vitamin D Analogues. Kidney International 78:134–139

Fish oils for kidney disease?

The omega-3 fatty acids, found abundantly in fish oils, seem to have much to offer the patient in kidney failure. In addition to reducing generalized inflammation in a variety of tissues and organs including the kidney, and thereby offering some protection against further decline, fish oils may even help the kidney transplant patient prevent organ rejection. Papers that discuss these issues at length are as follows:

—**Reddy VS, Dakshinamurty KV, Sherke RL, Parsad TN** 2002 Omega-3 Polyunsaturated Fatty Acids in the Prevention of Progression of Chronic Renal Disease. Indian Journal of Nephrology 12:6–9

—**Garman JH, Mulroney S, Maniqrasso M, Flynn E, Maric C** 2009 Omega-3 Fatty Acid Rich Diet Prevents Diabetic Renal Disease. Am J Physiol Renal Physiol 296:F306–F316

—**Hassan IR, Gronert K** 2009 Acute Changes in Dietary ω-3 and ω-6 Polyunsaturated Fatty Acids have a Pronounced Impact on Survival following Ischemic Renal Injury and Formation of Renoprotective Docosahexaenoic Acid-Derived Protectin D1. The Journal of Immunology 182:3223–3232

—**Simopoulos AP** 2002 Omega-3 Fatty Acids in Inflammation and Autoimmune Diseases. Journal of the American College of Nutrition 21(6):495–505

On a related note

Higher vitamin D levels are associated with a decreased risk of pelvic floor disorders in women. (Balalian and Rosenbaum, 2010)

There are several lines of evidence suggesting a potential role of vitamin D in the development of BPH [benign prostatic hyperplasia]. (Manchanda et al., 2012)

Now that we are going to all the trouble of saving your kidneys, we'd better make sure you can pee normally. Vitamin D may help.

In ladies, chronic vitamin D deficiency predisposes to problems associated with voiding. It leads to muscular weakness and what is called pelvic floor dysfunction. Pelvic floor dysfunction can, in turn, lead to stress urinary incontinence (SUI) and urgency urinary incontinence (UUI). You live in fear of your next sneeze, or you are constantly on the lookout, making sure a restroom is nearby.

Regarding pelvic floor dysfunction, I have two case reports to share.

> The first case was a 78-year-old female with UUI symptoms who had vitamin D deficiency [25(OH)D = 10 ng/ml]. She used 50,000 IU of vitamin D_2 twice monthly for one year, and then 100,000 IU/month for another year prior to being seen. Her repeat 25(OH)D after this prolonged supplementation was 21 ng/ml. She was treated with 50,000 IU of vitamin D_2 weekly for 6 months with improvement of her 25(OH)D to 54 ng/ml. The patient reported resolution of her UUI had resolved and she no longer wore protective pads. The second reported case was a 59-year-old female with SUI symptoms who had a 25(OH)D level of 13 ng/ml. She was given 50,000 IU of vitamin D_2 supplementation weekly for 12 weeks and her vitamin D level was increased to 43 ng/ml after 6 weeks. At her 3 month follow-up she reported resolution of her symptoms. (Parker-Autry et al., 2012)

In gentlemen, prostate enlargement, known clinically as benign prostatic hyperplasia (BPH), causes men to stand around a lot, and strain, while waiting for something favorable to happen (like voiding). Vitamin D deficiency can contribute to this disease process, and for a variety of reasons. Its ability to promote normal growth patterns is certainly one of them (Manchanda et al., 2012). One vitamin D analog, given the name BXL628, shows great promise in *"arresting the growth"* of the enlarged prostate (Manchanda et al., 2012; Colli et al., 2006). Recall from a previous discussion, vitamin D in various forms binds its receptor, the VDR, and initiates favorable genetic responses like promoting normal growth patterns. So, it stands to reason *"VDR has emerged as a vital factor in BPH . . . . Therefore, to ignore the connotation of VDR and its potential impact on morbidity and mortality in the BPH patient is no longer appropriate."* (Manchanda et al., 2012) Pretty strong words!

There is another hideous problem that many gentlemen face as they get older (also related to waiting for something favorable to happen). Erectile dysfunction appears more likely in the setting of prolonged vitamin D deficiency (Sorenson and Grant, 2012). Here, protection against vascular disease and dysfunction appears to be the protective effect offered by vitamin D in this situation. Combine cigarette smoking (which also lowers vitamin D levels) with hypovitaminosis D, and you could find yourself paying a lot more attention to certain TV commercials.

Chapter 21
Areas of controversy and concern

Despite evidence of its <u>profound</u> importance to human health, vitamin D deficiency is not widely recognized as a problem by physicians and patients. ~**Holick, 2006a, emphasis added**

*The American Academy of Dermatology recommends that an adequate amount of vitamin D should be obtained from a healthy diet that includes foods naturally rich in vitamin D, foods/beverages fortified with vitamin D, and/or vitamin D supplements. **Vitamin D should not be obtained from unprotected exposure to ultraviolet (UV) radiation.*** ~**American Academy of Dermatology, 2009, emphasis added**

*Some dermatologists advise that people of all ages and ethnicities should avoid all direct exposure to sunlight and should always use sun protection when outdoors. **This message is not only unfortunate, it is misguided and has serious consequences**, i.e., the risk of vitamin D deficiency. There is <u>little evidence</u> that adequate sun exposure will substantially increase the risk of skin cancer, rather, long-term excessive exposure and repeated sunburns are associated with nonmelanoma skin cancers.* ~**Holick, 2003, emphasis added**

The 30-year campaign of recommending abstinence from sun exposure has not decreased the incidence of nonmelanoma skin cancer or melanoma, but it has promoted vitamin D deficiency. ~**Holick, 2008**

When the Institute of Medicine (IOM) of the National Academies released its new Dietary Reference Intakes for Calcium and Vitamin D report on 30 November 2010, the vitamin D research community was shocked and dismayed at the findings. ~**Grant, 2011**

C learly, there is disagreement among the experts, and on some very important matters. You need to be aware of this and realize that not everybody has read *The Impact of Vitamin D Deficiency*. Therefore, you will be faced with a variety of opinions and actions related to a physician's level of understanding and beliefs regarding the issues we have discussed in the pages of this book.

Obviously, if you receive clear medical advice to avoid sun exposure or to limit or avoid vitamin D supplementation, by all means carefully consider the recommendation. Since there are some medical conditions that do require one to be very careful with sunlight exposure and vitamin D supplementation, following such advice may be a good call. But for the rest of us . . . *no exposure to sunlight!!?* And *just enough vitamin D to squeak by!!?* I'm not sure this is the advice that we should be receiving. I, along with many others, believe that we as a society are in the midst of an epidemic of vitamin D deficiency, and in order to gain the upper hand, sunlight exposure and vitamin D supplementation should be encouraged. I and many others believe that sunlight exposure and vitamin D supplementation can both be safely done with limited health risk. We will discuss the precautions, caveats, and recommendations of sunlight exposure and vitamin D supplementation in the following two chapters. Now back to controversies and concerns.

Due to an increased risk of skin cancer—particularly high under certain circumstances—sunlight exposure is strongly discouraged by many, notably by those within the Dermatology community. Accordingly, sunscreen is aggressively promoted to prevent skin cancer from UVB radiation exposure, leaving us to rely on Plan B and Plan B alone when it comes to achieving and maintaining vitamin D sufficiency. On the other hand, there are many others of equal caliber who believe there is little risk of skin cancer if sunlight exposure is practiced within reason (no sunburning or overexposure), believing that sunlight avoidance is an unfortunate teaching, one that will perpetuate vitamin D deficiency in our population. They may also be of the belief that vitamin D judiciously derived from the sun or by diet and supplementation may actually protect against skin cancer (Holick,

2006b; Holick, 2005; Bikle, 2009). Then there is the issue of vitamin D supplementation and how much is required.

Many believe that we as a society are basically sufficient in vitamin D, with an intake of 400, 800, even 1,000 IU/day certainly being enough to satisfy the needs of the average individual—based on the belief that rickets is no longer a major issue today and that there is little evidence that vitamin D has value beyond bone health and mineral balance. Yet, on the other hand, many others of equal caliber believe we need much higher levels of vitamin D than are usually considered "sufficient," levels where we begin to see a real difference in health and disease prevention. And so the D-bate continues.

Then there is the IOM.

> Numerous studies have reported an inverse association with vitamin D status, i.e., lower serum 25-hydroxyvitamin D (25[OH]D) levels are associated with increased risk of cancers of the breast, prostate, and colon among others; type 2 diabetes; cardiovascular disease; multiple sclerosis; rheumatoid arthritis; osteoarthritis; preeclampsia; cesarean delivery; depression; Alzheimer's disease; infectious diseases; and neurocognitive dysfunction. However, **because these studies were association and observational studies, they were dismissed by the recent Institute of Medicine (IOM) report** on dietary reference intakes as not qualifying as a high enough level of evidence to confirm the beneficial effect of vitamin D on these nonskeletal-related health outcomes. (Holick, 2011, emphasis added)

Periodically, the best and the brightest are brought together to discuss the issues that are facing medicine, in a gathering called the Institute of Medicine (IOM). The conclusions reached then become the standard of practice for others to follow. In 2010 the IOM was convened in order to hammer out issues related to vitamin D and calcium requirements. The results were not pleasing, at least not to those at the forefront of vitamin D research, nor to loveable guys writing vitamin D books in the corner of their living room.

To be brief, the IOM looked at the research, excluded studies that were "observational" in nature, and came to the conclusion that Americans are getting enough vitamin D from their current level of intake and current level of sunlight exposure. This conclusion, as one might expect, took the vitamin D research community by complete surprise. To say the least, there was great disappointment felt not only by the vitamin D research community but also by physicians, those who had been paying close attention to vitamin D in their everyday clinical practice. I believe the words "shocked" and "dismayed" were used to describe the reaction by the vitamin D experts to the report issued by the IOM. Obviously the IOM did not read *The Impact of Vitamin D Deficiency*, or the results would have been totally different. How unfortunate.

And speaking of unfortunate, as a result of the IOM report many a physician, looking for guidance, is being dissuaded from paying close attention to vitamin D. Furthermore, lab tests for routine screening of vitamin D deficiency are now being actively discouraged. And, silently, the epidemic continues. But what about Charlie?

You read about Charlie in *Chapter 18* and are still deeply concerned. He is at risk for some very bad things. And there is little Jimmy, little Billie, and little Suzie's friend Sarah. Will they go the way of the indoor people?—shielded from the sun and given only enough vitamin D to squeak by?

And what about the elderly, what about those in pain, what about the risk of cancer, and what about autoimmunity, what about diabetes, what about the challenge of obesity, what about those with darker skin, what about those who may become pregnant, what about . . . . So many diseases have been "observed" to occur far less frequently in those who are vitamin D sufficient yet prey on those who are deficient. There is strong scientific evidence as to why this is so. Vitamin D is a hormone that clearly influences the performance of cells and promotes a vast array of favorable responses.

Let's end this chapter with the words of a professor of Dermatology, one of great standing, one with over 100 peer-reviewed publications bearing his name. He must be very smart, perhaps wise. Maybe he can help put things into perspective.

In conclusion, dermatologists and other physicians have to be aware that strict sun protection to prevent skin cancer may induce the severe health risk of vitamin D deficiency. To guarantee a sufficient vitamin D status, dermatological recommendations on sun protection and health campaigns for skin cancer prevention will have to be re-evaluated. There is no doubt that UV radiation is mutagenic and is the main reason for the development of non-melanoma skin cancer. Therefore, excessive sun exposure has to be avoided, particularly burning in childhood. To reach this goal, the use of sunscreens as well as the wearing of protective clothes and glasses is absolutely important. Additionally, sun exposure around midday should be avoided during the summer in most latitudes. However, the dermatological community has to recognize that there is convincing evidence that the protective effect of less intense solar radiation outweighs its mutagenic effect. In consequence, **many lives could be prolonged through careful exposure to sunlight or more safely, vitamin D supplementation, especially in non-summer months.** (Reichrath, 2007, emphasis added)

Read all about it!

You can read the 700 page IOM 2010 report and try to figure out what was going through their heads, or you can read the responses made by the vitamin D experts. It's your choice.

A summary of the IOM report can be found at:

—**Brief Report: Dietary Reference Intakes for Calcium and Vitamin D**
www.iom.edu/Reports/2010/Dietary-Reference-Intakes-for-Calcium-and-Vitamin-D/Report-Brief.aspx

The best papers in opposition to the IOM report are as follows:

—Heaney RP, Holick MF 2011 Why the IOM Recommendations for Vitamin D are Deficient. Journal of Bone and Mineral Research 26(3):455–457

—Holick MF, Binkley NC, Bischoff-Ferrair HA, Gordon CM, Hanley DA Heaney RP, Murad MH, Weaver CM 2012 Guidelines for Preventing and Treating Vitamin D deficiency and Insufficiency Revisited. J Clin Endocrino Metab; April; 97(4):1153–1158

—Holick MF 2012 Evidence-Based D-Bate on Health Benefits of Vitamin D Revisited. Dermato-Endocrinology; April/May/June; 4(2):183–190

The following papers are in support of the IOM report on calcium and vitamin D. (Don't bother.)

—Szmuilowicz ED, Manson JE 2011 How Much Vitamin D Should You Recommend to your Nonpregnant Patients? OBG Management; July; 23(7):44–53

—Ross AC, Manson JE, Abrams SA, Aloia JF, Brannon PM, Clinton SK, Durazo-Arvizu RA, et al 2011 The 2011 Report on Dietary Reference Intake for Calcium and Vitamin D from the Institute of Medicine: What Clinicians Need to Know. J Clin Endocrinol Metab; January; 96(1):53–58

—Aloia JF The 2011 Report on Dietary Reference Intake for Vitamin D: Where Do We Go From Here? J Clin Endocrinol Metab; October; 96(10):2987–2996

—Abrams SA 2013 Dietary Guidelines for Calcium and Vitamin D: A New Era. Pediatrics; March; 127(3):566–568

Loose ends

There are a couple more quotations that I wanted to share with you in this chapter, but I couldn't figure out how to fit them in. Then the thought occurred to me, "Why not place them in the gray box at the end of the chapter?" This, of course, this was a great idea. They are good quotes, and you need to read them.

> The widespread concern about any direct sun exposure increasing the risk of the relatively benign and nonlethal squamous and basal cell cancers needs to be put into perspective. It is chronic excessive exposure to sunlight and sunburning experiences during childhood that increases risk of nonmelanoma skin cancer. Melanoma, one of the most feared cancers because of its ability to rapidly metastasize before it is obvious to either the patient or physician, has been branded as a sun-induced skin cancer. However, **most melanomas occur on the least sun-exposed areas**, and it has been reported that occupational exposure to sunlight decreases risk of melanoma. (Holick, 2006b, emphasis added)

And,

> Individuals are constantly told not to receive direct sun exposure or to wear sunscreen if they do. By following this advice, we are eliminating the initial step in an important endocrine system that can easily generate 10,000–20,000 IU/d vitamin D. How do we compensate for this? It is not likely with an intake of 400 IU/d vitamin D. Other confounding factors include dark skin pigmentation and northern latitudes, which inhibit cutaneous vitamin D3 production. We are rapidly becoming completely dependent on dietary supplementation as a means to ensure adequate vitamin D concentrations, and 400 IU/d is far from adequate. Second, maternal intake of 400 IU/d vitamin D does not elevate the nutritional status of mothers or nursing infants. This is indicated by the occurrence of hypovitaminosis D and rickets among breastfed infants. Maternal intake of 2,000 IU/d vitamin D elevates maternal 25(OH)D concentrations, but the amount passed on to nursing infants through the milk is still inadequate to elevate the infants' circulating 25(OH)D concentrations satisfactorily. Maternal intake of 4,000 IU/d increases maternal circulating concentrations to a degree that enough vitamin D enters the milk to produce significant effects on the infants' circulating 25(OH)D concentrations. (Hollis and Wagner, 2004)

The areas of controversy and concern discussed in this chapter and in this gray box will certainly be debated for some time, if not forever. But you don't have forever. You and your physician have many things to consider when deciding which course of action to take when it comes to sunlight exposure and vitamin D supplementation. Or you can go the way of the indoor people. It's your choice.

Chapter 22
Be safe out there . . . please!

Studies among normal adults demonstrate that oral vitamin D intakes of up to 10,000 IU/d for a period of 5 mo are safe, with no evidence of toxicity. **~Hollis and Wagner, 2004**

Thus, it was concluded that ***a daily intake of 10,000 IU should be considered the tolerable upper intake level.*** *There is no known medical reason for dosages approaching that level; hence, there is a comfortable margin of safety between therapeutic and toxic intakes.* **~Heaney, 2008, emphasis added**

Hypervitaminosis D is usually associated with prolonged exposure to very high doses of vitamin D (e.g., >10,000 IU/d), with a number of case reports documenting vitamin D toxicity from frequent ingestion of supplements containing very high amounts of vitamin D. Excessive sunlight or exposure to tanning beds does not cause vitamin D toxicity because prolonged UV light exposure degrades vitamin D precursors, preventing excessive formation of vitamin D_3. **~Krasowski, 2011, emphasis added**

We've talked a little about safety here and there as we have journeyed together through the pages of this book, but not nearly enough. Now we will focus on safety (while we can still focus). First off, I want to strongly emphasize the importance of avoiding sunburning. But, unfortunately, there is a certain degree of risk in practically everything you do, and sun-related damage to the skin, over time, is simply a fact of life. But you don't need to burn or be overexposed to the sun to get plenty of vitamin D in the intended way, and you can and <u>should</u> use sunscreen to prevent sunburning in a program that allows you to get vitamin D per sunlight exposure. As far as sun vs. skin goes, the weight of the evidence strongly suggests that our need for vitamin D outweighs the risks of sunlight exposure, at least most of the time. Without sufficient sunlight exposure, the risk of many diseases (some that can kill you) goes way up, unless you supplement adequately or have an unusual diet rich in vitamin D. (In which case, I will miss all the walruses you will be eating).

Since the skin is the organ that manufactures vitamin D for us, free of charge, we should probably let it perform this service whenever it is feasible. Due to the limited amount of vitamin D in our diet, unless you supplement in generous amounts, you will probably be deficient if you habitually avoid sunlight exposure, particularly during the time of day (10 AM to 3 PM, mid spring to early fall) when UVB rays are available to accomplish this task. It's that simple.

In all of this there are a few safety rules for you to keep in mind. What follows is supported by the literature but may not be the view of your physician or the medical community as a whole. I'm still working on them, but, at the moment, they are not impressing me. None of what follows is complicated.

The **first rule** of safety is to not get sunburned, period. **Period!** Are we clear? After a reasonable amount of sunlight exposure, say 15 minutes to a maximum of 30 minutes (sooner if exposed to intense sunlight), the use of sunscreen is a good call. Aside from protecting against sunburning, should you chose the right kind of sunscreen—one that also blocks UVA rays—you can also protect yourself against hideous wrinkles (Misra et al., 2008). UVA rays penetrate deeper than UVB rays, and therefore may be more damaging, at least more damaging than previously thought.

Perhaps the **second rule** would be not to take vitamin D in excess. This is why testing is in order. I don't care if you have to pay for it should your insurance company not cover the cost of the 25OHD test. Testing is very important. It will determine how pathetic your vitamin D level really is. Repeated testing will determine if treatment is effective and your approximate daily need for vitamin D.

The **third rule** is to go slowly at first with vitamin D supplementation. I and others believe that prescribing the "rescue" high-dose vitamin D_2 protocol (i.e., 50,000 IU/week x 8 to 12 weeks) is not always the best course of action. If this approach is offered to you, a good alternative to suggest would be 10,000 IU/day of D_3 for a trial period of several weeks, retest, and then go from there. It may be wise to go slowly at first, with perhaps 1,000 to 2,000 IU/day for a week or two, just to see if you tolerate vitamin D in increased amounts. We have previously discussed a number of medical conditions that warrant caution with vitamin D supplementation (see gray box at the end of *Chapter 5*), so be particularly careful if you fit into this category.

The **fourth rule** is to stop supplementation <u>immediately</u> should you experience any unusual symptom or an increase in disease activity, particularly if you have a chronic illness that you are grappling with. Contact your physician if you believe you are having trouble with vitamin D supplementation.

The **fifth rule** just makes sense. Re-test periodically throughout the year (and particularly after completion of a high-dose treatment regimen). At the very least get tested during winter to see if you are at a level your physician feels comfortable with. Unless you are faithful supplementing with vitamin D, and adequately supplementing, a normal vitamin D level in the fall will not mean that your level will be normal during winter and the following spring.

The **sixth rule** is to take enough vitamin D to do the job. Re-testing is the key here. Some studies suggesting that vitamin D supplementation makes no difference in certain disease states may be flawed due to the fact that the treated group is simply not given enough vitamin D to do the trick.

The **seventh rule** is something my personal physician shared with me. Find a vitamin D supplement of good quality (Hint: not the cheapest) and stick with it. Apparently, not all vitamin D supplements act the same even if the IUs are supposed to be identical. Therefore, if a brand switch occurs, subsequent testing may misinform and make it more difficult to properly prescribe further dosing. By way of example:

If you have a vitamin D level of 52 and you are advised to continue on the 6,000 IU/d, as previously ordered, should you now switch brands, your vitamin D level may drop to, say, 34 and not be at a level the physician is particularly pleased with. (My physician wants my level to be over 50.) I actually had this experience. Taking vitamin D is not rocket science, but it seems reasonable to stick with one brand and one form so that testing throughout the year will produce more reliable data. Another thing to keep in mind: If you switch from D_3 to D_2, a drop in your vitamin D level, too, may occur. And, may I add, D_3 has been shown to be a better choice than D_2 (Armas et al., 2004).

The **eighth rule**: In the summer, and on the summer days you get plenty of sunshine exposure between the hours of 10 AM and 3 PM, you should be able to miss a few days of taking vitamin D supplements. Your excellent, vitamin D-savvy physician will advise you—you have one, right? This brings us to the ninth rule.

The **ninth rule** is one that just I made up, but is certain to find favor with those in the forefront of vitamin D research. This rule states that if your physician is not all that into vitamin D, you must find one who is. Or you have some convincing to do. Hey, why not purchase an extra copy of this book and give it to your physician as a gift? Wrap it up and pretend it's for his or her birthday.

Safety is undoubtedly a concern with any medication. And, yes, I want you to consider your vitamin D supplement as medication. Clearly, the best approach is to have professional help to make sure you are doing things right. Today, with the availability of 25OHD2 testing, vitamin D supplementation can be tailored to individual need, and it can be done safely.

Since it seems as though anything that has rules should have at least ten of them to make things sound complete, I guess I'll have to make up one more safety rule.

The **tenth rule** states: If any rule shows up that I did not mention here you can follow it as long as it is a good rule, is simple, and makes perfect sense.

Problems in the past

In the 1950s an unfortunate outbreak of vitamin D intoxication occurred in England, related to an industrial mistake that occurred during the fortification of milk with vitamin D. Consequently, in England the D-fortification of milk was and remains prohibited by law (Holick, 2010). This reaction is actually a tragedy, continually placing this population at greater risk of vitamin D deficiency (and disease, suffering, and untimely death).

There are several individual cases of vitamin D intoxication on record; however, vitamin D intoxication is, thankfully, a rare occurrence. It is estimated that your vitamin D level would need to approach 150 ng/ml for vitamin D toxicity to occur. One would have to be very aggressive with vitamin D supplementation in order to reach that level unless certain circumstances exist. Doses of vitamin D up to 10,000 IU/day are generally regarded as safe, even by those who feel that supplementation is generally not necessary. (see Heaney 2008; Holick, 2011) In fact, 50,000 IU/week of vitamin D_2 is often prescribed for a period of 8 to 12 weeks. And although intolerance does occur, this practice does not seem to lead to toxicity.

Chapter 23
Recommendations

As mentioned earlier, health professionals need to "broaden their horizon" and think of vitamin D in more global health terms that incorporate vitamin D's true role as a hormone. The vitamin D endocrine system is the <u>only</u> steroid endocrine system in the body that is almost always limited by substrate [stuff to work with] availability because of latitude, life-style, race/skin pigmentation, sunlight exposure, and other factors. **~Wagner et al., 2008, emphasis added**

Vitamin D deficiency and its consequences are extremely subtle, but have <u>enormous</u> implications for human health and disease. It is for this reason that vitamin D deficiency continues to go unrecognized by a majority of health professionals. **~Holick, 2003a, emphasis added**

A minimum concentration of 25(OH)D should be 50 nmol/L [20 ng/ml], and, for maximum bone health and prevention of many chronic diseases, the 25(OH)D concentration should be 78–100 nmol/L [31–40 ng/ml]. **~Holick, 2004a**

L et's make this vitamin D thing easy (sort of). Again, I'll rely on the advice of the experts, the ones who eat, sleep, and breathe vitamin D. Warning: I'll need to pack a lot of information in here, but take things point by point and you won't get lost. (But if you do get lost, we'll send someone out to find you. Just don't get too lost.) I will also make clever little headings to help hold your interest. I am that nice. What follows are the recommendations, with a few exceptions, gleaned directly from the medical literature. Consider the following:

- **Help is on the way**

    Invite your physician to read this book! Place it in his or her hands because you have never seen such a compelling book on vitamin D—so funny and cleverly written, too! Sure, you can get vitamin D supplements over the counter and self-medicate, but to do things right, you need a physician on board (one who knows this stuff or is willing to learn and practice . . . on you!). Don't assume that your physician is up to speed on vitamin D issues. Little of this is taught in med school, leaving physicians to learn the ins and outs of vitamin D all on their own. The gift of this book may help. You can explain the tough parts, if need be.

- **Shoot for this**

    The vitamin D level believed (by the experts) to be ideal is between 40 to 60 ng/ml. Above this range, there appears to be little in the way of added benefit (according to the experts), although there are always some exceptions. In some cases, large amounts of vitamin D supplementation may be required, but not for the average individual.

- **Can I take too much vitamin D? (Yes, of course you can.)**

    But don't fall for statements such as: "You can get too much vitamin D from sunlight!" And, "Following the 3,000–6,000 IU/d recommendation may be dangerous, perhaps crazy!" *Old school!* Even those who downplay the need to supplement above what is required to maintain bone integrity will admit that 10,000 IU/d is a safe amount (under most circumstances) (Holick, 2011). However, there are some very important exceptions: You may not tolerate a high-dose vitamin D regimen (i.e., 50,000 IU of vitamin D_2 once a week for 8 to 12 weeks, a regimen often given to "rescue" individuals from a very low vitamin D status). This is why having a vitamin D-savvy physician comes in very handy in determining the best course of action to take. Additionally, there is a concern that higher doses of vitamin D will lead to higher calcium levels and may, therefore, lead to the formation of kidney stones. This may be an important consideration in a certain subset of individuals, but not in everyone. Your doctor may have this legitimate concern. You may want to listen!

- **How much do I need?**
  "It has been estimated that the body requires daily 3,000 to 5,000 IU of vitamin D." (Holick, 2005, emphasis added) And if you are pregnant or nursing you may need up to **6,000 IU/day**, possibly more! (Hollis, 2007; Hollis and Wagner, 2006) Bottom line: 3,000 IU to 6,000 IU is probably not too much for the average individual to take, but get tested just to make sure that you are taking the right amount and not taking vitamin D in excess. *"Unless a 25 (OH)D level is determined, it is impossible to know if a person is sufficient in vitamin D. Further, symptoms of vitamin D deficiency are very subtle and often go undetected."* (Holick, 2002)

- **Seriously ill?**
  A 25(OH)D$_3$ level is fine for screening purposes. But if you are dealing with a serious disease, a disease like Crohn's or even rheumatoid arthritis, insist on having a 1,25(OH)$_2$D$_3$ level drawn, too—it may yield other clues as to what is going on inside. In Crohn's disease, the 1,25(OH)$_2$D$_3$ level may be elevated and cause harm, remember? In rheumatoid arthritis, low levels of 1,25(OH)$_2$D$_3$ might be found and be a clinically important finding (Arnson et al., 2007).

- **Regarding tanning beds**
  Tanning beds may or may not help you improve your vitamin D status (Holick, 2005). They need to be *UVB-emitting* tanning beds, not the more common *UVA-emitting* tanning

beds, in order to generate vitamin D within the skin (Koutkia et al., 2001). The use of a UVB tanning bed has been recommended in cases when there is a malabsorption syndrome in play, one that is preventing the absorption of vitamin D from the gut (Holick, 2004a). Tanning beds work! (see Tangpricha et al., 2004) But be careful! You can "sunburn" in a tanning bed.

- **What about cancer?**

    Check to see if vitamin D supplementation may interfere with a certain therapeutic approach that you may be undertaking (i.e., chemotherapy)—very possible, particularly with respect to Hodgkin's and non-Hodgkins lymphoma. Of particular concern is the tendency for hypercalcemia to develop, due to the unregulated $1,25(OH)_2D_3$ production common to these two cancers (Tuohy and Steinman, 2005). Things get even more complicated due to the fact that chemotherapy is associated with a lowering of vitamin D levels (Fakih et al., 2009). So it behooves the physician to be up to speed on the issues related to cancer, cancer therapy, and vitamin D, in as much as vitamin D is involved in many physiological processes related to the development and progression of cancer. That being said—due to the complex nature of cancer—it behooves the cancer patient to be careful with vitamin D supplementation and not supplement without physician approval and close monitoring.

- **I can't believe how big I have become (on that darn Western diet)!**

    If you are significantly overweight, become very serious about vitamin D. Fat cells are very good at storing vitamin D. This "reservoir" needs filled up before you can hope to become vitamin D sufficient on an ongoing basis and be able to provide other organs and systems with their fair share of vitamin D

(DeLuca, 2004; Holick, 2004a). One low lab result addressed by an 8-week course of *mega-dose* vitamin D will not suffice (Holick, 2004b). A regimen of 50,000 IU vitamin D every other week (Holick, 2005), or perhaps once a month (Holick, 2002; Holick, 2003b) until vitamin D levels are normalized has been recommended. If low vitamin D levels persist, a "rescue," high dose vitamin D regimen as often as every 3 to 6 months (Lee et al., 2008) may be necessary until you achieve satisfactory results and maintain a respectable level of vitamin D. Bottom line: *Do not* settle for anything less than ongoing vitamin D sufficiency, overweight or not. Do what it takes to achieve a vitamin D level that you can brag about! Bragging rights probably begin at 50 ng/ml. But remember, you may have to settle for less under certain medical circumstances.

- **Winter has rolled around, once again**

    Live in fear of winter (unless you're prepared). Be aware that winter increases your need for Plan B. Due to the angle of the sun, during winter little if any vitamin D will be obtained via Plan A. During wintertime especially, supplementation with adequate amounts of vitamin D is a must. If consuming 5 to 10 cans of tuna *and* 20 to 30 glasses of fortified orange juice per day seems a little unreasonable, try taking a dietary supplement.

- **Measuring up**

    "*Annual measurements of serum 25(OH)D is a reasonable approach to monitoring for vitamin D deficiency.*" (Holick, 2004a) Of course, treat low vitamin D levels to achieve and maintain 25(OH)D within the latest recommendations. Hint: "*There is growing evidence that circulating 25OHD levels >40 ng/ml are necessary to achieve full physiologic vitamin D actions.*" (Zittermann et al., 2003)

- **Making sense out of it all**

     Practice *sensible* sunlight exposure. *Seriously* avoid sun burning and being baked to death in the desert by the sun. (Try to prevent being boiled to death, too—only invites cannibalism! So often I issue this warning.) Take special precautions if you have a vulnerable skin type or red hair (natural red hair). Use sunscreen wisely. Join a nudist camp. (Well, it's a thought!—perhaps the board of directors will let you mow the lawn). If you are regularly exposed to sunlight, you should be able to limit your oral intake of vitamin D supplements, tuna, etc. Just don't be overexposed or get sunburned. Are we clear?

- **Tan without really trying**

     If you have a dark skin complexion, your skin type is especially adapted to tolerate (and require) more sunlight exposure, making you a special target for vitamin D deficiency—particularly so if you live in the northern hemisphere and are one of those darn indoor people. You need to pay special attention to the issue of dietary supplementation, as casual sunlight exposure will just not be effective. It has been estimated that black-skinned people need up to **10 times** more sunlight exposure to generate the same vitamin D levels as the light-skinned individual (Dawodu and Wagner, 2007).

- **This is *huge*!**

     Some individuals may not tolerate the "mega-dose" approach to correcting a low vitamin D level (like my dear mother). Consider this:

     Hypersensitivity to vitamin D can occur. Primary hyperparathyroidism is probably the most common example. . . . In hyperparathyroid individuals, vitamin D exaggerates hypercalcemia because of the connection between vitamin D and $1,25(OH)_2D$ production. (Vieth, 1999)

Should hypersensitivity be a concern or pop up out of nowhere, start or resume supplementation using regular-strength vitamin D, at a low dose, and then gradually increase your daily intake of vitamin D as tolerated, under your doctor's supervision of course. (The physician should review Norman, 2008, for an alternative approach to the use of "mega-dose" D_2. His recommendation is to abandon the 50,000 IU/d D_2 method, believing that a high-dose D_3 regimen is a more physiologic approach. Other sources suggest upwards to 10,000 IU/d of D_3 (the typical form of supplemental vitamin D) may be in order until normal vitamin D levels are restored. This level of supplementation is believed to be generally safe (Giovannucci, 2009; Khan and Fabian, 2010).

- **You're special!**

  Persons with unusual medical conditions like **sarcoidosis**, **tuberculosis**, or **lymphoma** may be advised not to try to increase their vitamin D level at all! (Veith, 1999; Tuohy and Steinman, 2005; Schwalfenberg, 2007)

> **The most serious side effect of vitamin D treatment is hypercalcemia, which itself <u>can be lethal</u>. Therefore, caution is warranted in the use of vitamin D as a treatment for MS, RA, and IDDM [insulin dependent diabetes mellitus], but so is further investigation into the possible connections between vitamin D status and autoimmune diseases.** (Cantorna, 2000, emphasis added)

See, if you are dealing with a serious medical condition, you will need professional care in managing hypovitaminosis D. *I'm dead serious!* Even with professional care, if you are on a prescribed, mega-dose *"rescue"* vitamin D_2 program and you seem to be having unusual or distressing symptoms, stop therapy <u>immediately</u> and call your physician. A new strategy may be in order. Reacting to vitamin D is a serious matter. It can happen! It can be bad.

- **Do not try *this* at home**

    Do *not* try to increase your vitamin D level by increasing your daily-multivitamin intake. **Wrong move!** This may lead to excessive increases of vitamin A. And if you are pregnant this can *increase in the risk of birth defects.* In others, this can increase in the risk of osteoporosis (Holick, 2004a).

- **Do not try *this* any longer**

    Smoking (and possibly second-hand smoking) can lower vitamin D levels (Brot et al., 1999); so can alcohol abuse (Laitinen and Välimäki, 1991). You probably don't need either of these. Both can ruin your life (in many, many ways). You're cool enough.

- **Got drugs?**

    Certain drugs can lower vitamin D levels. These include **Fosamax** and **Actonel** (Mann, 2005); **anticonvulsants** like **Dilantin and Phenobarbital, corticosteroids** [e.g., **prednosone**], and **Questran** (Holick, 2006); **Plaquenil**, a drug used to treat both lupus (Huisman et al., 2001) and rheumatoid arthritis (*Web*MD, 2008); and drugs that do not improve a patient's vitamin D status **because they are not vitamin D!** (I thought this last one up all on my own.)

- **It's what's inside that matters**

    There is some concern that certain preparations of vitamin D may have ingredients that affect the bioavailability of the vitamin itself (Leventis and Patel, 2008). Perhaps. If your vitamin D supplement does not seem to improve your vitamin D status as anticipated, this may be an important consideration.

Switch brands, or consider that your replacement dose is just not adequate.

- **Something just ain't right**

    Having a problem tolerating supplemental vitamin D? I am aware that some people cannot seem to tolerate the vitamin D that comes in the usual, oil-filled softgel. They can, however, sometimes do well with a dry, granular formulation placed in a typical gelatin capsule. And sometimes individuals can tolerate D_2 when they cannot tolerate D_3.

- **Is now a good time?**

    One report suggests that in order to get the maximum effect from your vitamin D supplement, take it with your biggest meal of the day. I make all my meals the biggest meal of the day, so I am a little bit confused here. (see Mulligan and Licata, 2010)

What is a safe upper level of vitamin D?

That all depends on you! You are a different person. (I mean this in a way slightly different than others do whenever your name comes up.) The fact is, *everyone* has a unique chemistry and has a different set-point of physiologic need. This is why everyone should be tested to see where they are at, and then be retested periodically to see if they are right on track or at least headed in the right direction. Some people, to their surprise, find that in spite of eating 5 to 10 cans of tuna a day, they are still deficient in vitamin D. And some people, to everyone's surprise, discover that their vitamin D level is actually "undetectable!" If this were to happen to you, you might hear the words, "And you're still alive?"

On the other end of the spectrum, some people have what may seem to be too high of a vitamin D level. So let's listen to what the experts have to say. I have two in mind:

At the present time, 25(OH)D levels in the range of 30 to 60 ng/ml are considered optimal, but higher levels up to 100 ng/ml are often seen in individuals with outdoor occupations receiving intense sun exposure without ill effects.

Vitamin D intoxication with renal stones and hypercalcemia may be observed when serum levels of 25(OH)D are greater than 150 ng/mL (374 nmol/L). For a good margin of safety, levels greater than 100 ng/mL should probably be avoided. (Khan and Fabian, 2010)

When is too much too much?

Answer: When it is too much! We have discussed certain conditions where vitamin D therapy may have to be limited or not pursued at all, such as sarcoidosis and certain forms of cancer. But should you be alarmed if you are placed on a high dose of vitamin D? Generally not. (Okay, for some of you, just go ahead and worry about this, too!) Again, let's turn to the experts:

Vitamin D, particularly its active hormonal form, calcitriol, is a highly potent molecule, capable of producing serious toxic effects, including death, at milligram intake levels. There is thus a healthy fear of the compound relating in part to cases of sporadic poisoning as well as to medical misadventure 70 years ago, involving administration of millions of units per day of the vitamin. Nevertheless, despite these appropriate concerns there is in fact, a comfortable margin of safety between the intakes required for optimization of vitamin D status and those associated with toxicity. It is worth noting that, for example, a single minimum erythema [skin] dosage of ultraviolet radiation (e.g., 15 min in the sun in a bathing suit in July) produces, in a light-skinned individual, 10,000 to 20,000 IU of vitamin D. Repeated day after day, this can add up to substantial vitamin D inputs. Nevertheless, there has never been a reported case of vitamin D intoxication from sun exposure. Controlled metabolic studies, necessarily limited in scope (although expanding into the 100s of individuals), showed that dosages up to 50,000 IU/d for from 1–5 months produce neither hypercalcemia nor hypercalciura [high calcium in bloodstream or in urine]. A recent publication, reviewing the reported for daily intakes of <30,000 IU/d for extended periods and no cases of vitamin D intoxication for serum 25(OH)D levels <200 ng/ml (500 nmol/L). Thus, it was concluded that a daily intake of 10,000 IU should be considered the tolerable upper intake level. There is no known medical reason for dosages approaching that level; hence, there is a comfortable margin of safety between therapeutic and toxic intakes. (Heaney, 2008, emphasis added)

Conclusion

Vitamin D deficiency and its consequences are extremely subtle, but have <u>enormous</u> implications for human health and disease. **~Holick, 2003, emphasis added**

Perhaps one of the greatest gifts medical science has to offer us today is the knowledge of what we can accomplish should we start paying close attention to the vitamin that is really a hormone. **~The Author, 2014**

C ongratulations! You've made it through the book . . . well, almost. Now you have a brief little *Conclusion* to finish. But I'm not even sure that a *Conclusion* is necessary at this point, now that you are totally convinced that vitamin D deficiency is, indeed, a setup for disease, suffering, tragedy, and untimely death. On the other hand, I'm sure we can find some unfinished business around here somewhere that we need to wrap up.

I read somewhere that a good book conclusion should summarize the important points previously presented, as well as motivate the reader to act. Mentioning disease, suffering, tragedy, and untimely death is probably enough of a summary of the important points we have discussed in the pages of this book. Now, how best to get you motivated? I guess I'll just have to scare you a little; it has worked before! Another brief discussion on cancer should do the trick.

We've read this before:

A more recent analysis estimated that currently between 50,000–63,000 Americans and 19,000–25,000 individuals living in

the United Kingdom annually die prematurely from cancer due to vitamin D deficiency. (Spina et al., 2006, emphasis added)

And we read this:

A pooled analysis of studies that assessed serum 25D in relation to breast cancer demonstrated a clear dose-response relationship, with the highest quintile [upper one fifth] of serum 25D associated with a **50% reduction in breast cancer risk.** (Welsh, 2007, emphasis added)

And you remember reading this:

Chronic vitamin D deficiency may have serious adverse consequences, including increased risk of hypertension, multiple sclerosis, cancers of the colon, prostate, breast, and ovary, and type 1 diabetes. (Holick, 2003)

(I know when to back off. I've scared you enough. . . . Well perhaps not. I don't see you trembling.)

Speaking of breast cancer: **In the United States, breast cancer alone kills more than 40,000 individuals per year!** (Cui and Rohan, 2006) **Yet vitamin D sufficiency may reduce this level of carnage, perhaps by half!** (Welsh, 2007) Are we paying attention? But it is not just death that we are dealing with here. There are multitudes of breast cancer patients who will survive but will never, *ever* be the same. Mastectomies are so commonplace in the world that I live in. I am reminded of this repeatedly in my nursing practice. (You won't like a mastectomy.) I am also reminded (repeatedly) of other cancers that can be prevented to a considerable extent by a life sufficient in vitamin D. Colon cancer readily comes to mind. Its rate, too, could be cut in half if our population were vitamin D sufficient. But we are not. But we should be. But we are not.

There are a whole host of diseases besides cancer that increase in frequency in those who are deficient in vitamin D. You've heard of

Parkinson's disease and Alzheimer's disease. You've heard of MS. You've heard of cardiovascular disease, including heart attack and stroke. You've heard of Crohn's disease and collection bags that never go away. And you've heard of damaged children, brought into this world vitamin D deficient and facing life-long challenges such as autism and schizophrenia. (I could go on and on, but I will spare you.) Clearly, there would be less disease, suffering, tragedy, and untimely death if hypovitaminosis D were rare rather than the norm.

But look at me—dwelling on the negative. I actually have some good news to share!

There are many physicians who practice medicine who believe and are up to speed on the issues related to vitamin D. They have recognized the significance of what the science has been saying for years, even decades! And they are acting, not waiting for committees to speak or for directives to be handed down. As a result, patients are being successfully treated for their vitamin/hormone deficiency, and *exceptional* results are being seen. Some call their results **"remarkable"** (Al Faraj and Al Matairi, 2003). Lives are being transformed! Diseases are being prevented! Body parts are being spared! Wheelchairs are for sale on eBay! Loveable guys writing vitamin D books in the corner of their living room are happy, but not happy enough. They still see disease, suffering, tragedy, and untimely death occurring in the context of an epidemic that should not exist and is more evil than one can imagine. They also seek clever little ways of bringing a book to a close.

I sincerely hope that you were paying close attention during the few hours we have spent together. My goal was to share with you the impact of vitamin D deficiency on the lives of people like you and people like me and motivate you to act. In all of this, I have done my very best to share with you what this vitamin D business is all about and to help you forget about the plight of Gilligan, at least for a while. I would still worry about Charlie.

I leave you with this:

Vitamin D deficiency requires immediate attention and aggressive vitamin D replacement. (Holick, 2008)

But, perhaps, I can have the last word:

You don't actually die from hypovitaminosis D itself, it just makes it easier for other things to kill you! (The Author, 2014, emphasis added)

~Acknowledgments~

I wish to thank the following people who helped make this book possible: First and foremost, my dear wife Toni, whose support and encouragement has helped make this book a reality. I extend a special thanks to Gail Leong and Sandy Keno, both medical librarians at Providence Sacred Heart, Spokane, Washington. These two librarians are indoor people (I am trying to save them both). I also wish to think my editor and proofreader, Jacquelyn Barnes. Her job was not an easy one.

~Appendix~

Conversion Formulas

They're not making it easy on us, are they? Sometimes lab results and research literature list vitamin D concentrations in nmol/L instead of the usual ng/ml that shows up on the laboratory report. Not only that, the dose of vitamin D given in a particular clinical trial may be listed in micrograms instead of IUs. Here is an example: If your vitamin D level is 50 nmol/l, sounds good, but don't start bragging. Your vitamin D level is actually 20 ng/ml—way too low. Your physician is alarmed (and so am I), realizing that you have been squeaking by only on 10 µgs of vitamin D/day. You are now wisely placed on 100 µgs of vitamin D/day. This means you were taking a pitiful 400 IU/day, but your luck has changed! Your doctor has now placed you on a more realistic dose of vitamin D, 4,000 IU/day.

Here are the conversion formulas that will help you sort everything out:

- To convert to nmol/L to ng/ml, multiply nmol/L by 0.4. Example: 35 nmol/L x 0.4 = 14 ng/ml.

- To convert mcg's (µgs) to International Units (IU), multiply mcg x 40. Example: 25 µgs x 40 = 1,000 IU.

Recommended websites

There are several websites well worth recommending. Here are my favorites:

- *Vitamin D Council.* **www.vitamindcouncil.org**

- *Pain Treatment Topics.* **www.pain-topics.org**

- *Vitamin D Health.org.* **www.vitamindhealth.org**

- *The Impact of Vitamin D Deficiency* official website (accept no substitutes). **www.impactofvitamind.com**

~References~

Introduction

DeLuca H 2004 Overview of General Physiological Features and Functions of Vitamin D. Am J Clin Nutr 80(Suppl):1689S–1696S

Holick MF 2002 Vitamin D: The Unappreciated D-lightful Hormone that is Important for Skeletal and Cellular Health. Current Opinion in Endocrinology & Diabetes 9:87–98

Holick MF 2003 Vitamin D: A Millenium Perspective. Journal of Cellular Biochemistry 88:296–307

Holick MF 2004a Vitamin D: Importance in the Prevention of Cancers, Type 1 Diabetes, Heart Disease, and Osteoporosis. American Journal of Clinical Nutrition; March; 79(3):362–371

Holick MF 2004b Sunlight and Vitamin D for Bone Health and Prevention of Autoimmune Diseases, Cancers, and Cardiovascular Disease. American Journal of Clinical Nutrition; December; 80(6):1678S–1688S

Holick MF 2006 High Prevalence of Vitamin D Inadequacy and Implications for Health. Mayoclinicproceedings.com

Hollis BW, Wagner Cl 2006 Vitamin D Requirements during Lactation: High-Dose Maternal Supplementation as Therapy to Prevent Hypovitaminosis D for Both the Mother and the Nursing Infant. Am J Clin Nutr 80(Suppl):1752S–1758S

Chapter 1 (Natural history)

Cekic M, Cutler SM, VanLandingham JW, Stein DG 2011 Vitamin D Deficiency Reduces the Benefits of Progesterone Treatment after Brain Injury in Aged Rats. Neurobiology of Aging 32:864–874

Holick MF 2003 Vitamin D: A Millenium Perspective. Journal of Cellular Biochemistry 88:296–307

Chapter 2 (Basics, briefly)

Adorini L, Penna G 2008 Control of Autoimmune Diseases by the Vitamin D Endocrine System. Nature Clinical Practice Rheumatology; August; 4(8):404–412

Cui Y, Rohan TE 2006 Vitamin D, Calcium, and Breast Cancer Risk: A Review. Cancer Epidemiol Biomarkers Prev 15(18):1427–1437

DeLuca H 2004 Overview of General Physiological Features and Functions of Vitamin D. Am J Clin Nutr 80(Suppl):1689S–1696S

Eyles D, Brown J, MacKay-Sim A, McGrath J, Feron F 2003 Vitamin D and Brain Development. Neuroscience 118:641–653

Ginde AA, Mansbach JM, Camago CA 2009 Association Between Serum 25-Hydroxyvitamin D Level and Upper Respiratory Tract Infection in the Third National Health and Nutrition Examination Survey. Arch Intern Med 169(4)384–390

Heaney RP 2003 Long-Latency Deficiency Disease: Insights from Calcium and Vitamin D. Am J Clin Nutr 78:912–919

Holick MF 2002 Vitamin D: The Unappreciated D-lightful Hormone that is Important for Skeletal and Cellular Health. Current Opinion in Endocrinology & Diabetes 9:87–98

Holick MF 2004a Vitamin D: Importance in the Prevention of Cancers, Type 1 Diabetes, Heart Disease, and Osteoporosis. American Journal of Clinical Nutrition; March; 79(3):362–371

Holick MF 2004b Sunlight and Vitamin D for Bone Health and Prevention of Autoimmune Diseases, Cancers, and Cardiovascular Disease. American Journal of Clinical Nutrition; December; 80(6):1678S–1688S

Holick MF 2005 The Vitamin D Epidemic and its Health Consequences. J. Nutr. 135:2739S–2748S

Holick MF 2006a High Prevalence of Vitamin D Inadequacy and Implications for Health. Mayoclinicproceedings.com

Holick MF 2006b Resurrection of Vitamin D Deficiency and Rickets. The Journal of Clinical Investigation 116(16):2062–2072

Holick MF 2007 Vitamin D Deficiency. N Engl J Med; July 19; 357:266–281

Holick MF 2008 Vitamin D: A D-Lightful Health Perspective. Nutrition Reviews 66(Suppl 2):S182–S194

Lappe JM, Travers-Gustafson D, Davies KM, Recker RR, Heaney RP 2007 Vitamin D and Calcium Supplementation Reduces Cancer Risk: Results of a Randomized Trial. Am J Clin Nutr 85:1586–1591

McCann JC, Ames BN 2008 Is There Convincing Biological of Behavior Evidence Linking Vitamin D Deficiency to Brain Dysfunction? FASEB 22:982–1001

Miller Jr DW 2007 Vitamin D in a New Light. http://archive.lewrockwell.com/miller/miller25.html

Nakanishi-Matsui M, Kashiwagi S, Hosokawa H, Cipriano DJ, Dunn SD, Wada Y, Futai M 2006 Stochastic High-Speed Rotational of *Escherichia coli* ATP Syntase F1 Sector. Journal of Biological Chemistry; February; 281(7):4126–4131

Peterlik M, Cross HS 2005 Vitamin D and Calcium Deficits Predispose for Multiple Chronic Diseases. European Journal of Clinical Investigation 35:290–304

Sato Y, Asoh T, Kondo I, Satoh K 2001 Vitamin D and Risk of Hip Fractures Among Disabled Elderly Stroke Patients. Stroke 32:1673–1677

Shin JS, Shoi MY, Longtine MS, Nelson MN 2010 Vitamin D Effects on Pregnancy and the Placenta. Placenta 31(12):1027–1034

Spina CS, Tangpricha V, Uskokovic M, Adorinic L, Maehr H, Holick MF 2006 Vitamin D and Cancer. Anticancer Research 26:2515–2524

Steingrimsdottir L, Gunnarsson O, Indridason OS, Franzson L, Sigurdsson G 2005 Relationship Between Serum Parathyroid Hormone Levels, Vitamin D Sufficiency, and Calcium Intake. JAMA; November 9; 294(18):2336–2341

Sutton AL, MacDonald PN 2003 Vitamin D: More Than a "Bone-a-Fide" Hormone. Molecular Endocrinology 17(5):777–791

Schwartz M 2002 Autoimmunity as the Body's Defense Mechanism Against the Enemy Within: Development of Therapeutic Vaccines for Neurodegenerative Disorders. Journal of NeuroVirology 8:480–485

VanAmerongen BM, Dijkstra CD, Lips P, Polman CH 2004 Multiple Sclerosis and Vitamin D: An Update. European Journal of Clinical Nutrition 58:1095–1109

Vieth R 1999 Vitamin D Supplementation, 25-hydroxyvitamin D Concentrations, and Safety. American Journal of Clinical Nutrition 69(5):842–856

Wagner CL, Taylor SN, Hollis BW 2008 Does Vitamin D Make the World Go "Round"? Breastfeeding Medicine 3(4):239–250

Whitton PS 2007 Inflammation as a Causative Factor in the Aetiology of Parkinson's Disease. Br J Pharmacol; April; 150(8)963–976

Zittermann A 2003 Vitamin D in Preventive Medicine: Are We Ignoring the Evidence? British Journal of Nutrition 89:552–572

Chapter 3 (Action at the nuclear level)

Bolland MJ, Avenell A, Baron JA, Grey A, MacLennan GS, Gamble GD, Reid IR 2010 Effect of Calcium Supplements on Risk of Myocardial Infarction and Cardiovascular Events: Meta-analysis. BMJ 341: doi:10.1136/BMJ.c3691

Cui Y, Rohan TE 2006 Vitamin D, Calcium, and Breast Cancer Risk: A Review. Cancer Epidemiol Biomarkers Prev 15(18):1427–1437

Holick MF 2002 Vitamin D: The Unappreciated D-lightful Hormone that is Important for Skeletal and Cellular Health. Current Opinion in Endocrinology & Diabetes 9:87–98

Holick MF 2003 Vitamin D Deficiency: What a Pain It Is. Mayo Clin Proc 78:1457–1459

Holick MF 2004a Vitamin D: Importance in the Prevention of Cancers, Type 1 Diabetes, Heart Disease, and Osteoporosis. American Journal of Clinical Nutrition; March; 79(3):362–371

Holick MF 2004b Sunlight and Vitamin D for Bone Health and Prevention of Autoimmune Diseases, Cancers, and Cardiovascular Disease. American Journal of Clinical Nutrition; December; 80(6):1678S–1688S

Holick MF 2006 Resurrection of Vitamin D Deficiency and Rickets. The Journal of Clinical Investigation 116(16):2062–2072

Holick MF 2007 Vitamin D Deficiency. N Engl J Med; July 19; 357:266–281

Kamimura S, Gallieni M, Zhong M, Beron W, Slatopolsky E, Dusso A 1995 Microtubules Mediate Cellular 25-Hydroxyvitamin D_3 Trafficking and the Genomic Response to 1,25-Dihydroxyvitamin D_3 in Normal Human Monocytes. The Journal of Biological Chemistry; September 22; (38):22160–22166

Lappe JM, Travers-Gustafson D, Davies KM, Recker RR, Heaney RP 2007 Vitamin D and Calcium Supplementation Reduces Cancer Risk: Results of a Randomized Trial. Am J Clin Nutr 85:1586–1591

Miller Jr DW 2007 Vitamin D in a New Light. LewRocknwll.com

Peterlik M, Cross HS 2005 Vitamin D and Calcium Deficits Predispose for Multiple Chronic Diseases. European Journal of Clinical Investigation 35:290–304

Spina CS, Tangpricha V, Uskokovic M, Adorinic L, Maehr H, Holick MF 2006 Vitamin D and Cancer. Anticancer Research 26:2515–2524

Sutton AL, MacDonald PN 2003 Vitamin D: More Than a "Bone-a-Fide" Hormone. Molecular Endocrinology 17(5):777–791

VanAmerongen BM, Dijkstra CD, Lips P, Polman CH 2004 Multiple Sclerosis and Vitamin D: An Update. European Journal of Clinical Nutrition 58:1095–1109

Vieth R 1999 Vitamin D Supplementation, 25-hydroxyvitamin D Concentrations, and Safety. American Journal of Clinical Nutrition 69(5):842–856

Wagner CL, Taylor SN, Hollis BW 2008 Does Vitamin D Make the World Go "Round"? Breastfeeding Medicine 3(4):239–250

Wikipedia 2010 DNA Repair. http://en.wikipedia.org/wiki/DNA_repair

Chapter 4 (You're not getting enough)

Hayes CE, Cantorna MT, DeLuca HF 1997 Vitamin D and Multiple Sclerosis. P.S.E.B.M. 216:21–27

Holick MF 2002 Vitamin D: The Unappreciated D-lightful Hormone that is Important for Skeletal and Cellular Health. Current Opinion in Endocrinology & Diabetes 9:87–98

Holick MF 2004 Sunlight and Vitamin D for Bone Health and Prevention of Autoimmune Diseases, Cancers, and Cardiovascular Disease. American Journal of Clinical Nutrition; December; 80(6):1678S–1688S

Holick MF 2006a High Prevalence of Vitamin D Inadequacy and Implications for Health. Mayoclinicproceedings.com

Holick MF 2006b Resurrection of Vitamin D Deficiency and Rickets. The Journal of Clinical Investigation 116(16):2062–2072

Holick MF 2007 Vitamin D Deficiency. N Engl J Med; July 19; 357:266–281

Holick MF 2008 Vitamin D: A D-Lightful Health Perspective. Nutrition Reviews 66(Suppl 2):S182–S194

Kaushal M, Magon N 2013 Vitamin D in Pregnancy: A Metabolic Outlook. Indian J Endocrinol Metab; January–February; 17(1):76–82

Lee JH, O'Keefe JH, Bell D, Hensrud DD, Holick MF 2008 Vitamin D Deficiency: An Important, Common, and Early Treatable Cardiovascular Risk Factor. Journal of the American College of Cardiology 52(24):1949–1956

McGrath J, Saari K, Hakko H, Jokelainen J, Jones P, Järvelin M, Chant D, Isohanni M 2004 Vitamin D Supplementation During the First Year of Life and Risk of Schizophrenia: A Finish Birth Cohort Study. Schizophrenia Research 67:237–245

Peterlik M, Cross HS 2005 Vitamin D and Calcium Deficits Predispose for Multiple Chronic Diseases. European Journal of Clinical Investigation 35:290–304

Spina CS, Tangpricha V, Uskokovic M, Adorinic L, Maehr H, Holick MF 2006 Vitamin D and Cancer. Anticancer Research 26:2515–2524

VanAmerongen BM, Dijkstra CD, Lips P, Polman CH 2004 Multiple Sclerosis and Vitamin D: An Update. European Journal of Clinical Nutrition 58:1095–1109

Wagner CL, Taylor SN, Hollis BW 2008 Does Vitamin D Make the World Go "Round"? Breastfeeding Medicine 3(4):239–250

Chapter 5 (The price we are paying)

Adorini L, Penna G 2008 Control of Autoimmune Diseases by the Vitamin D Endocrine System. Nature Clinical Practice Rheumatology; August; 4(8):404–412

Fakih MG, Trump DL, Johnson CS, Tian L, Muindi J, Sunga AY 2009 Chemotherapy is Linked to Severe Vitamin D Deficiency in Patients with Colorectal Cancer. Int J Colorectal Dis 24:219–224

Holick MF 2003 Vitamin D: A Millenium Perspective. Journal of Cellular Biochemistry 88:296–307

Holick MF 2005 The Vitamin D Epidemic and Its Health Consequences. J. Nutr. 135:2739S–2748S

Holick MF 2006 High Prevalence of Vitamin D Inadequacy and Implications for Health. Mayoclinicproceedings.com

McCann JC, Ames BN 2008 Is there Convincing Biological of Behavior Evidence Linking Vitamin D Deficiency to Brain Dysfunction? FASEB 22:982–1001

Peterlik M, Cross HS 2005 Vitamin D and Calcium Deficits Predispose for Multiple Chronic Diseases. European Journal of Clinical Investigation 35:290–304

Schwalfenberg G 2007 Not Enough Vitamin D: Health Consequences for Canadians. Canadian Family Medicine 53:842–854

VanAmerongen BM, Dijkstra CD, Lips P, Polman CH 2004 Multiple Sclerosis and Vitamin D: An Update. European Journal of Clinical Nutrition 58:1095–1109

Wagner CL, Taylor SN, Hollis BW 2008 Does Vitamin D Make the World Go "Round"? Breastfeeding Medicine 3(4):239–250

Chapter 6 (Cancer)

Bläuer M, Rovio PH, Ylikomi T, Heinonen PK 2009 Vitamin D Inhibits Myometrial and Leiomyoma Cell Proliferation in Vitro. Fertility and Sterility 91(5):1919–1925

Grimes DS 2006 Are Statins Analogues of Vitamin D? Lancet 368:83–86

Holick MF 2003 Vitamin D: A Millenium Perspective. Journal of Cellular Biochemistry 88:296–307

Holick MF 2004a Vitamin D: Importance in the Prevention of Cancers, Type 1 Diabetes, Heart Disease, and Osteoporosis. American Journal of Clinical Nutrition; March; 79(3):362–371

Holick MF 2004b Sunlight and Vitamin D for Bone Health and Prevention of Autoimmune Diseases, Cancers, and Cardiovascular Disease. American Journal of Clinical Nutrition; December; 80(6):1678S–1688S

Holick MF 2006a High Prevalence of Vitamin D Inadequacy and Implications for Health. Mayoclinicproceedings.com

Holick MF 2006b Resurrection of Vitamin D Deficiency and Rickets. The Journal of Clinical Investigation 116(16):2062–2072

Holick MF 2007 Vitamin D Deficiency. N Engl J Med; July 19; 357:266–281

Holick MF 2008 Vitamin D: A D-Lightful Health Perspective. Nutrition Reviews 66(Suppl 2):S182–S194

Lappe JM, Travers-Gustafson D, Davies KM, Recker RR, Heaney RP 2007 Vitamin D and Calcium Supplementation Reduces Cancer Risk: Results of a Randomized Trial. Am J Clin Nutr 85:1586–1591

Mariani E, Ravaglia G, Forti P, Meneghetti A, Tarozzi A, Maioli F, Boschi F, Pratelli L, Pizzoferrato A, Piras F, Facchini A 1999 Vitamin D, Thyroid Hormones and Muscle Mass Influence Natural Killer (NK) Innate Immunity in Healthy Nonagenarians and Centarians. Clin Exp Immunol; April; 116(1):1–27

Spina CS, Tangpricha V, Uskokovic M, Adorinic L, Maehr H, Holick MF 2006 Vitamin D and Cancer. Anticancer Research 26:2515–2524

Sutton AL, MacDonald PN 2003 Vitamin D: More Than a "Bone-a-Fide" Hormone. Molecular Endocrinology 17(5):777–791

Welsh J 2007 Vitamin D and Prevention of Breast Cancer. Acta Pharmacol Sin; September; 28(9):1373–1382

Chapter 7 (Diabetes)

American Association of Diabetes Educators 2012 AADE Position Statement: Diabetes and Physical Activity. American Association of Diabetes Educators; January/February; 38(1)129–132

DeLuca H 2004 Overview of General Physiological Features and Functions of Vitamin D. Am J Clin Nutr 80(Suppl):1689S–1696S

Fernández-Real JM, López-Bernejo A, Richart W 2002 Cross-Talk Between Iron and Diabetes. Diabetes 51:2348–2354

Hill JO, Wyatt HR, Reed GW, Peters JC 2003 Obesity and the Environment: Where Do We Go from Here? Science; February 7; 299:853–855

Holick MF 2002 Vitamin D: The Unappreciated D-lightful Hormone that is Important for Skeletal and Cellular Health. Current Opinion in Endocrinology & Diabetes 9:87–98

Holick MF 2006 Resurrection of Vitamin D Deficiency and Rickets. The Journal of Clinical Investigation 116(16):2062–2072

Holick MF 2007 Vitamin D Deficiency. N Engl J Med; July 19; 357:266–281

Jiang R, Manson JE, Meigs JB, Ma J, Rifai N, Hu FB 2004 Body Iron Stores in Relation to Risk of Type 2 Diabetes in Apparently Healthy Women. JAMA; February 11; 291(6):711–717

Martínez-Garcia MA, San-Millán JL, Luque-Ramírez M, Escobar-Morreale HF 2009 Body Iron Stores and Glucose Intolerance in Postmenopausal Women. Diabetes Care 32(8):1525–1530

Mathieu C, Badenhoop K 2005 Vitamin D and Type 1 Diabetes Mellitus: State of the Art. Trends in Endocrinology and Metabolism; August; 16(6):261–265

Munger KL, Levin LI, Hollis BW, Howard NS, Ascherio A 2006 Serum 25-Hydroxyvitamin D Levels and Risk of Multiple Sclerosis. JAMA; December 20; 296(23):2832–2838

Peterlik M, Cross HS 2005 Vitamin D and Calcium Deficits Predispose for Multiple Chronic Diseases. European Journal of Clinical Investigation 35:290–304

Pittas AG, Lau J, Hu FB, Dawson-Hughes B 2007 The Role of Vitamin D and Calcium in Type 2 Diabetes. A Systematic Review and Meta-Analysis. The Journal of Endocrinology & Metabolism 92(6):2017–2029

Pradhan AD, Manson JE, Rifai N, Buring JE, Ridker PM 2001 C-Reactive Protein, Interleukin 6, and Risk of Developing Type 2 Diabetes Mellitus. JAMA; July 18; 286(3):327–334

Zella JB, DeLuca HF 2003 Vitamin D and Autoimmune Diabetes. Journal of Cellular Biochemistry 88:216–222

Chapter 8 (Autoimmune disease)

Ackerman D 2007 Hypercalcemia in Sarcoidosis—Case Report, Prevalence, Pathophysiology and Therapeutic Options. Ther Umsch; May; 64(5):281–286

Adorini L, Penna G 2008 Control of Autoimmune Diseases by the Vitamin D Endocrine System. Nature Clinical Practice Rheumatology; August; 4(8):404–412

Arnson Y, Amital H, Shoenfeld Y 2007 Vitamin D and Autoimmunity: New Aetiological and Therapeutic Considerations. Ann Rheum Dis; June 8; 0:1–6

Barnes TC, Bucknall RC 2004 Vitamin D Deficiency in a Patient with Systemic Lupus Erthematosus. Rheumatology 43:393–394

Boccaccio GL, Steinman L 1996 *Mini-Review* Multiple Sclerosis: From a Myelin Point of View. Journal of Neuroscience Research 45:647–654

Cantorna MT, Hayes CE, DeLuca H 1998 1,25-Dihydroxycholecalciferol Inhibits the Progression of Arthritis in Murine Models of Human Arthritis. J. Nutr. 128:68–72

Cantorna MT 2008 Vitamin D and Multiple Sclerosis: An Update. Nutrition Reviews 66(Suppl 2):S135–S138

Chaudhuri A 2005 Why We should Offer Routine Vitamin D Supplementation in Pregnancy and Childhood to Prevent Multiple Sclerosis. Medical Hypotheses 64:608–618

Cutolo M, Otsa K, Uprus M, Paolino S, Seriolo B 2007 Vitamin D in Rheumatoid Arthritis. Autoimmunity Reviews 7:59–64

Durmus B, Altay Z, Baysal O, Ersoy Y 2012 Does Vitamin D Affect Disease Severity in Patients with Ankylosing Spondylitis? Chin Med J 125(14):2511–2515

Franco PG, Silvestroff L, Soto EF, Pasquini GM 2008 Thyroid Hormones Promote Differentiation of Oligodendrocyte Progenitor Cells and Improve Remyelination after Cuprizone-Induced Demyelination. Experimental Neurology 212:458–467

Ginanjar E, Sumariyono, Setiati S, Setiyohadi B 2007 Vitamin D and Autoimmune Disease. Acta Med Indones-Indones J Intern Med; July–September; 39(3):133–141

Hayes CE 2000 Vitamin D: A Natural Inhibitor of Multiple Sclerosis. Proceedings of the Nutrition Society 59:531–535

Hayes CE, Cantorna MT, DeLuca HF 1997 Vitamin D and Multiple Sclerosis. P.S.E.B.M. 216:21–27

Hayes CE, Nashold FE, Spach KM, Pedersen LB 2003 The Immunological Functions of the Vitamin D Endocrine System. Cell. Mol. Biol. 49(2):1–24

Holick MF 2004 Sunlight and Vitamin D for Bone Health and Prevention of Autoimmune Diseases, Cancers, and Cardiovascular Disease. American Journal of Clinical Nutrition; December; 80(6):1678S–1688S

Holick MF 2005 The Vitamin D Epidemic and Its Health Consequences. J. Nutr. 135:2739S–2748S

Holick MF 2006 Resurrection of Vitamin D Deficiency and Rickets. The Journal of Clinical Investigation 116(16):2062–2072

Islam T, Gauderman WJ, Cozen W, Mack TM 2007 Childhood Sun Exposure Influences Risk of Multiple Sclerosis in Monozygotic Twins. Neurology 69:381–388

Kelly C, Hamilton J 2006 What Kills Patients with Rheumatoid Arthritis? Rheumatology 46:183–184

Lanza FL, Chan FK, Quigley EM 2009 Guidelines for Prevention of NSAID-Related Ulcer Complications. The American Journal of Gastroenterology; March; 104:728–738

Leventis P, Pater S 2008 Clinical Aspects of Vitamin D in the Management of Rheumatoid Arthritis. Rheumatology 47:1617–1621

Mathieu C, Badenhoop K 2005 Vitamin D and Type 1 Diabetes Mellitus: State of the Art. Trends in Endocrinology and Metabolism; August; 16(6):261–265

McTigue DM, Tripathi RB 2008 The Life, Death, and Replacement of Oligodendrocytes in the Adult CNS. Journal of Neurology 107(1):1–19

Orton S, Morris AP, Herrera BM, Ramagopalan SV, Lincoln MR, Chao MJ, Vieth R, Sadovnick AD, Ebers GC 2008 Evidence for Genetic Regulation of Vitamin D Status in Twins with Multiple Sclerosis. Am J Clin Nutr 88:441–447

Potera C 2009 Vitamin D Regulates MS Gene. Environ Health Perspect; May; 117(5):A196

Ruiz-Irastorza G, Egurbide MV, Olivares N, Martinez-Berriotxoa A, Aguirre C 2008 Vitamin D Deficiency in Systemic Lupus Erythematosus: Prevalence, Predictors and Clinical Consequences. Rheumatology 47:920–923

Spach KM, Pedersen LB, Nashold FE, Kayo T, Yandell BS, Prolla TA, Hayes CE 2004 Gene Expression Analysis Suggests that 1,25-Dihydroxyvitamin D3 Reverses Experimental Autoimmune Encephalomyelitis by Stimulating Inflammatory Cell Apotosis. Physiol Genomics 18:141–151

VanAmerongen BM, Dijkstra CD, Lips P, Polman CH 2004 Multiple Sclerosis and Vitamin D: An Update. European Journal of Clinical Nutrition 58:1095–1109

Zittermann A 2003 Vitamin D in Preventive Medicine: Are We Ignoring the Evidence? British Journal of Nutrition 89:552–572

Chapter 9 (IBD)

Abreu MT, Kantorovich V, Vasiliauskas EA, Gruntmanis U, Matuk R, Daigle K, Chen S, et al 2004 Measurement of Vitamin D Levels in Inflammatory Bowel

Disease Patients Reveals a Subset of Crohn's Patients with Elevated 1,25-Dihydroxyvitamin D and Low Mineral Density. Gut 53:1129–1136

Blanck S, Aberra F 2013 Vitamin D Deficiency is Associated with Ulcerative Colitis Disease. Dig Dis Sci; January; [Epub ahead of print]

Cantorna MT, Zhu Y, Froicu M, Wittke A 2004 Vitamin D Status, 1,25-Diydroxyvitamin D3, and the Immune System. Am J Clin Nutr 80(Suppl):1717S–1720S

Carroll ME, Schade DS 2003 A Practical Approach to Hypercalcemia. American Family Physician; May 1; 67(9):1959–1966

Cutolo M, Otsa K, Uprus M, Paolino S, Seriolo B 2007 Vitamin D in Rheumatoid Arthritis. Autoimmunity Reviews 7:59–64

Holick MF 2007 Vitamin D Deficiency. N Engl J Med; July 19; 357:266–281

Kelsall BL 2008 Innate and Adaptive Mechanisms to Control Pathological Intestinal Inflammation. J Pathol 214:242–259

Kong J, Zhang Z, Musch MW, Ning G, Sun J, Hart J, Bissonnette M, Li YC 2008 Novel Role of the Vitamin D Receptor in Maintaining the Integrity of the Intestinal Mucosal Barrier. Am J Physiol Gastrointest Liver Physiol 294:G208–G216

Liu N, Nguyen L, Chun RF, Lagishetty V, Ren S, Wu S, Hollis B, et al 2008 Altered Endocrine and Autocrine Metabolism of Vitamin D in a Mouse Model of Gastrointestinal Inflammation. Endocrinology 149(10):4799–4808

Mayer L 2000 Epithelial Cell Antigen Presentation. Curr Opin Gastroenterol; November; 16(6):531–535

Johansson M EV, Holmén JM, Hansson GC 2010 The Two Mucus Layers of Colon are Organized by the MUC23 Mucin, whereas the Outer Layer is a Legislator of Host–Microbial Interactions. PNAS; March 5; 108(Suppl. 1):4659–4665

Johansson M EV, Holmén JM, Hansson GC 2011 The Two Mucus Layers of Colon are Organized by the MUC23 Mucin, whereas the Outer Layer is a Legislator of Host–Microbial Interactions. PNAS; March 5; 108(Suppl. 1):4659–4665

McGuckin MA, Eri R, Simms LA, Florin T HJ, Radford-Smith G 2009 Intestinal Barrier Dysfunction in Inflammatory Bowel Disease. Inflamm Bowel Dis 15(1):100–113

Nairz M, Schroll A, Sonnweber T, Weiss G 2010 The Struggle for Iron—a Metal at the Host–Pathogen Interface. Cellular Microbiology 12(12):1691–1702

Neish AS 2002 The Gut Microflora and Intestinal Epithelial Cells: A Continuing Dialogue. Microbes and Infection 4:309–317

Nerich V, Jantchou P, Boutron-Ruault M-C, Monnet E, Weill A, Vanbockstael V, Auleley G-R, et al 2011 Low Exposure to Sunlight is a Risk Factor for Crohn's Disease. Aliment Pharmacol Ther 33:940–945

Peyrin-Biroulet L, Oussalah A, Bigard M-A 2009 Crohn's Disease: The Hot Hypothesis. Medical Hypotheses 73:94–96

Schneider H, Braun A, Füllekrug J, Stremmer W, Ehehalt R 1010 Lipid Based Therapy for Ulcerative Colitis—Modulation of Intestinal Mucus Membrane Phospholipids as a Tool to Influence Inflammation. Int. J. Mol. Sci. 11:4149–4164

Schoultz I, Söderholm JD, McKay DM 2011 Is Metabolic Stress a Common Denominator in Inflammatory Bowel Disease? Inflamm Bowel Dis; September; 17(9):2008–2018

Schwalfenberg G 2007 Not Enough Vitamin D: Health Consequences for Canadians. Canadian Family Medicine 53:842–854

Sun J 2010 Vitamin D and Mucosal Immune Function. Curr Opin Gastroenterol; November; 26(6):591–595

Wang T-T, Dabbas B, Laperriere D, Bitton AJ, Soualhine H, Tavera-Mendoza LE, Sionne S, et al 2010 Direct and Indirect Induction by 1,25-Dihydroxyvitamin D_3 of the NOD2/Card15-Defensin β2 Innate Immune Pathway Defective in Crohn Disease. Journal of Biological Chemistry; January 22; 285(4):2227–2231

Yamamoto-Furusho JK, Korzenik JR 2006 Crohn's Disease: Innate Immunodeficiency? World J Gastroenterol; November 14; 12(42):6751–6755

Schwalfenberg G 2007 Not Enough Vitamin D: Health Consequences for Canadians. Canadian Family Medicine 53:842–854

Chapter 10 (Parkinson's)

Boban M, Modun D 2010 Urid Acid and Antioxidant Effects of Wine. Croatian Medical Journal 51(1):16–22

Chorley B 2008 Vitamin D Insufficiency Common in Parkinson's Disease. NIEHS Environmental Factor; November; http:www.niehs.nih.gov/news/newsletter/2008/November/vitamin-d.cfm

Evatt ML, DeLong MR, Khazai N, Rosen A, Triche S, Tangpricha V 2008 Prevalence of Vitamin D Insufficiency in Patients with Parkinson Disease and Alzheimer Disease. Arch Neurol; October; 65(10):1348–1352

Fernandez de Abreu DA, Eyles D, Féron F 2009 Vitamin D, a Neuro-immunomodulator: Implications for Neurodegenerative and Autoimmune Diseases. Psychoneuroendocrinology doi:10.1016/J.Psyneuen.2009.05.023:1–13

Garcion E, Wion-Barbot N, Montero-Menei CN, Berger F, Wion D 2002 New Clues about Vitamin D Function in the Nervous System. Trends in Endocrinology and Metabolism; April; 13(3):100–105

Hooper DC, Spitsin S, Kean RB, Champion JM, Dickson GM, Chaidhry I, Koprowski H 1998 Uric Acid, a Natural Scavenger of Peroxynitrite, in Experimental Allergic Encephalomyelitis and Multiple Sclerosis. Proc. Natl. Acad. Sci.; January; 95:675–680

Nelson DA, Paulson GW 2002 Idiopathic Parkinson's Disease(s) May Follow Subclinical Episodes of Perivenous Demyelination. Medical Hypotheses 59(6):762–769

Newmark HL, Newmark J 2007 Vitamin D and Parkinson's Disease—A Hypothesis. Movement Disorders 22(4):461–468

Sadrzadeh SM, Saffari Y 2004 Iron and Brain Disorders. Am J Clin Pathol 121(Suppl 1):S64–S70

Whitton PS 2007 Inflammation as a Causative Factor in the Aetiology of Parkinson's Disease. Br J Pharmacol; April; 150(8)963–976

Chapter 11 (Alzheimer's disease)

Annweiler C, Rolland Y, Schott AM, Blain H, Vellas B, Beauchet O 2011 Serum Vitamin D Deficiency as a Predictor of Incident Non-Alzheimer Dementias: A 7-Year Longitudinal Study. Dement Geriatr Cogn Discord 32:273–278

Buell JS, Dawson-Hughes B2008 Vitamin D and Neurocognitive Dysfunction: Preventing "D"ecline? Molecular Aspects of Medicine 29:415–422

Dickens AP, Land IA, Langa KM, Kos K, Llewellyn DJ 2011 Vitamin D, Cognitive Dysfunction and Dementia in Older Adults. CNS Drugs 26(8):629–639

Dwyer BE, Zacharski LR, Balestra DJ, Lerner AJ, Perry G, Zhu X, Smith MA 2009 Getting the Iron Out: Phlebotomy for Alzheimer's Disease? Medical Hypotheses; May; 72(5):504–509

Holmes C, Cunningham C, Zotova E, Woolford J, Dean C, Kerr S, Culliford D, Perry VH 2009 Systemic Inflammation and Disease Progression in Alzheimer's Disease. Neurology 73:768–774

Ito S, Ohtskuki S, Koitabashi Y, Murata S, Terasaki T 2011 1α25-Dihydroxy-vitamin D3 Enhances Cerebral Clearance of Human Amyloid-β Peptide(1-14) from Mouse Brain Across the Blood-Brain Barrier. Fluids and Barriers of the CNS 8(20)

Quốc Lu'o'ng KV, Nguyễ LTH 2011 The Beneficial Role of Vitamin D in Alzheimer's Disease. American Journal of Alzheimer's Disease & Other Dementias 26(7):511–520

Soni M, Kos K, Lang IA, Jones K, Melzer D, Llewellyn DJ 2012 Vitamin D and Cognitive Function. Scandinavian Journal of Clinical & Laboratory Investigation 72(Suppl 243):79–82

Chapter 12 (Infectious disease)

Adorini L, Penna G 2008 Control of Autoimmune Diseases by the Vitamin D Endocrine System. Nature Clinical Practice Rheumatology; August; 4(8):404–412

Bals R, Weiner DJ, Moscioni AD, Meegalla RL, Wilson JM 1999 Augmentation of Innate Host Defense by Expression of a Cathelicidin Antimicrobial A Peptide. Infection and Immunity; November; 67(11):6084–6089

Cannell JJ, Zasloff M, Garland CF, Scragg R, Giovannucci D 2008 On the Epidemiology of Influenza. Virology Journal 5(29):doi:10.1186/1743-422X-5-29

Cantorna MT 2000 Vitamin D and Autoimmunity: Is Vitamin D Status an Environmental Factor Affecting Autoimmune Disease Prevalence? Proceedings of the Society for Experimental Biology and Medicine 223:230–233

Ginde AA, Mansbach JM, Camago CA 2009 Association Between Serum 25-Hydroxyvitamin D Level and Upper Respiratory Tract Infection in the Third National Health and Nutrition Examination Survey. Arch Intern Med 169(4)384–390

Grayson R, Hewison M 2011 Vitamin D and Human Pregnancy. Fetal and Maternal Medicine Review 22(1):67–90

Hata TR, Kotol P, Jackson M, Nguyen M, Paik A, Udall D, Kanada K, Yamasaki K, Alexandrescu D, Gallo RJ 2008 Administration of Oral Vitamin D Induces Cathelicidin Production in Atopic Individuals. J Allergy Clin Immunol 122(4): 829–831

Hayes CE, Nashold FE, Spach KM, Pedersen LB 2003 The Immunological Functions of the Vitamin D Endocrine System. Cell. Mol. Biol. 49(2):1–24

Heaney RF 2008 Vitamin D in Health and Disease. Clin J Am Soc Nephrol 3:1535–1541

Holick MF 2008 Vitamin D: A D-Lightful Health Perspective. Nutrition Reviews 66(Suppl 2):S182–S194

Schmidt DR, Mangelsdorf DJ 2008 Nuclear Receptors of the Enteric Tract: Guarding the Frontier. Nutrition Reviews 66(Suppl 2):S88–S97

Segaert S, Siminart S 2008 The Epidermal Vitamin D System and Innate Immunity: Some More Light Shed on This Unique Photoendocrine System. Dermatology 217:7–11

Chapter 13 (Cardiovascular disease)

Balden R, Selvamani A, Sohrabji F 2012 Vitamin D Deficiency Exacerbates Experimental Stroke Injury and Dysregulates Ischemia-Induced Inflammation in Adult Rats. Endocrinology; March 9; doi:10.1210/en.2011–1783

Bolland MJ, Avenell A, Baron JA, Grey A, MacLennan GA, Gamble GD, Reid IR 2010 Effect of Calcium Supplements on Risk of Myocardial Infarction and Cardiovascular Events: Meta-analysis. BMJ; 341:c3691 doi:10.1136/BMJ.c3691

Holick MF 2006 Resurrection of Vitamin D Deficiency and Rickets. The Journal of Clinical Investigation 116(16):2062–2072

Lee JH, O'Keefe JH, Bell D, Hensrud DD, Holick MF 2008 Vitamin D Deficiency: An Important, Common, and Early Treatable Cardiovascular Risk Factor. Journal of the American College of Cardiology 52(24):1949–1956

MacDonald HB 2008 Dairy Nutrition: What We Knew Then to What We Know Now. International Dairy Journal 18:774–777

Pilz S, März W, Wellnitz B, Seelhorst U, Fahrleitner-Pammer A, Dimai HP Boehm BO, Dobnig H 2008 Association of Vitamin D Deficiency with Heart Failure and Sudden Cardiac Death in a Large Cross-Sectional Study of Patients Referred for Coronary Angiography. J Clin Endocrinol Metab 93:3927–3935

Wang L, Manson JE, Song Y, Sesso HD 2010 Vitamin D and Calcium Supplementation in Prevention of Cardiovascular Events. Ann Intern Med 152:315–323

Zittermann A 2003 Vitamin D in Preventive Medicine: Are We Ignoring the Evidence? British Journal of Nutrition 89:552–572

Zittermann A, Schleithoff SS, Tenderich G, Berthold HK, Körfer R, Stehle P 2003 Low Vitamin D Status: A Contributing Factor in the Pathogenesis of Congestive Heart Failure? J Am Coll Cardiol 41:105–112

Chapter 14 (Neurodevelopmental and psychiatric disorders)

Anglin RES, Samaan Z, Walter SD, McDonald SD 2013 Vitamin D Deficiency and Depression in Adults: Systematic Review and Meta-Analysis. The British Journal of Psychiatry. 202:100–107

Cannell JJ 2008 Autism and Vitamin D. Medical Hypotheses 70:750–759

Dunn JT, Delange F 2001 Damaged Reproduction: The Most Important Consequence of Iodine Deficiency. The Journal of Clinical Investigation 86(6):2360–2363

Eyles D, Brown J, MacKay-Sim A, McGrath J, Feron F 2003 Vitamin D and Brain Development. Neuroscience 118:641–653

Eyles D, Almeras L, Benech P, Patatian A, Mackay-Sim A, McGrath J, Féron F 2007 Developmental Vitamin D Deficiency Alters the Expression of Genes Encoding Mitochondrial, Cytoskeletal and Synaptic Proteins in the Adult Rat Brain. Journal of Steroid Biochemistery & Molecular Biology 103:538–545

Fernandez de Abreu DA, Eyles D, Féron F 2009 Vitamin D, a Neuro-immunomodulator: Implications for Neurodegenerative and Autoimmune Diseases. Psychoneuroendocrinology doi:10.1016/J.Psyneuen.2009.05.023:1–13

Féron F, Burne TH, Brown J, Smith E, McGrath JJ, Mackay-Sim A, Eyles DW 2005 Developmental Vitamin D_3 Deficiency Alters the Adult Rat Brain. Brain Research Bulletin 65:141–148

Gracion E, Wion-Barbot N, Montero-Menei CN, Berger F, Wion D 2002 New Clues about Vitamin D Functions in the Nervous System. Trends in Endocrinology & Metabolism 13(3):100–105

Holick MF 2008 Vitamin D: A D-lightful Health Perspective. Nutrition Reviews 66(Suppl 2):S182–S194

Llewellyn DJ, Langa KM, Lang IA 2009 Serum 25-Hydroxyvitamin D Concentration and Cognitive Decline. Journal of Geriatric Psychology 000(00):1–8

McCann JC, Ames BN 2008 Is there Convincing Biological of Behavior Evidence Linking Vitamin D Deficiency to Brain Dysfunction? FASEB 22:982–1001

McGrath J 2001 Does "Imprinting" with Low Prenatal Vitamin D Contribute to the Risk of Various Adult Disorders? Medical Hypotheses 56(3):367–371

McGrath JJ, Eyles DW, Pedersen CB, Anderson C, Ko P, Burne TH, Norgaard-Petersen B, et al 2010 Neonatal Vitamin D Status and Risk of Schizophrenia. Arch Gen Psychiatry 67(9):889–894

Taylor SN, Wagner CL, Hollis BW 2009 Vitamin D Deficiency in Pregnancy and Lactation and Health Consequences. Clinic Rev Bone Miner Metab 7:42–51

VanAmerongen BM, Dijkstra CD, Lips P, Polman CH 2004 Multiple Sclerosis and Vitamin D: An Update. European Journal of Clinical Nutrition 58:1095–1109

Chapter 15 (Muscles and bones)

Basha B, Rao DS, Han Z, Parfitt M 2000 Osteomalacia due to Vitamin D Depletion: A Neglected Consequence of Intestinal Malabsorption. Am J Med. 108:296–300

Bolland MJ, Avenell A, Baron JA, Grey A, MacLennan GS, Gamble GD, Reid IR 2010 Effect of Calcium Supplements on Risk of Myocardial Infarction and Cardiovascular Events: Meta-analysis. BMJ 341: doi:10.1136/BMJ.c3691

Haussler MR, Haussler CA, Bartik L, Whitfield GK, Hsieh J, Slater S, Jurutka PW 2008 Vitamin D Receptor: Molecular Signaling and Actions of Nutritional Ligands in Disease Prevention. Nutrition Reviews 66(Suppl 2):S98–S112

Heaney RP 2003 Long-Latency Deficiency Disease: Insights from Calcium and Vitamin D. Am J Clin Nutr 78:912–919

Holick MF 2002 Vitamin D: The Unappreciated D-lightful Hormone that is Important for Skeletal and Cellular Health. Current Opinion in Endocrinology & Diabetes 9:87–98

Holick MF 2003b Vitamin D Deficiency: What a Pain It Is. Mayo Clin Proc 78:1457–1459

Holick MF 2004b Sunlight and Vitamin D for Bone Health and Prevention of Autoimmune Diseases, Cancers, and Cardiovascular Disease. American Journal of Clinical Nutrition; December; 80(6):1678S–1688S

Holick MF 2006a Resurrection of Vitamin D Deficiency and Rickets. The Journal of Clinical Investigation 116(16):2062–2072

Holick MF 2006b High Prevalence of Vitamin D Inadequacy and Implications for Health. Mayoclinicproceedings.com

Holick MF 2007 Vitamin D Deficiency. N Engl J Med; July 19; 357:266–281

Holick MF 2008 Vitamin D: A D-Lightful Health Perspective. Nutrition Reviews 66(Suppl 2):S182–S194

Lee JH, O'Keefe JH, Bell D, Hensrud DD, Holick MF 2008 Vitamin D Deficiency: An Important, Common, and Early Treatable Cardiovascular Risk Factor. Journal of the American College of Cardiology 52(24):1949–1956

Lips P 2006 Vitamin D Physiology. Progress in Biophysics and Molecular Biology 92:4–8

Sutton AL, MacDonald PN 2003 Vitamin D: More Than a "Bone-a-Fide" Hormone. Molecular Endocrinology 17(5):777–791

Takasu H 2008 Anti-osteoclastogenic Action of Active Vitamin D. Nutrition Reviews 66(Suppl 2):S113–S115

Zittermann A 2003 Vitamin D in Preventive Medicine: Are We Ignoring the Evidence? British Journal of Nutrition 89:552–572

Chapter 16 (Aches, pains, mobility)

Al Faraj SA, Al Mutairi JA 2003 Vitamin D Deficiency and Chronic Low Back Pain in Saudi Arabia. Spine 28:177–179

Atherton K, Berry DJ, Parsons T, Macfarlane GJ, Power C, Hyppönen E 2009 Vitamin D and Chronic Widespread Pain in a White Middle-aged British Population: Evidence from a Cross-sectional Population Survey. Ann Rheum Dis 68:817–822

Ghose R 2004a Osteomalacia: Recovery of Bone Density. Journal of the New Zealand Medical Association; June 18; 117(1196)

Ghose R 2004b Sub-clinical Osteomalacia. Journal of the New Zealand Medical Association; August 20; 117(1200)

Gleurp H, Mikkelsen K, Poulsen L, Hass E, Overbeck S, Andersen H, Charles P, Eriksen EF 2000 Hypovitaminosis D Myopathy Without Biochemical Signs of Osteomalacic Bone Involvement. Calcif Tissue Int 66:419–424

Holick MF 2004 Sunlight and Vitamin D for Bone Health and Prevention of Autoimmune Diseases, Cancers, and Cardiovascular Disease. American Journal of Clinical Nutrition; December; 80(6):1678S–1688S

Holick MF 2005 The Vitamin D Epidemic and Its Health Consequences. J. Nutr. 135:2739S–2748S

Holick MF 2007 Vitamin D Deficiency. N Engl J Med; July 19; 357:266–281

Holick MF 2008 Vitamin D: A D-Lightful Health Perspective. Nutrition Reviews 66(Suppl 2):S182–S194

Mascarenhas CV, Mobarhan S 2004 Hypovitaminosis D-Induced Pain. Nutrition Reviews; September; 62(9):354–359

Plehwe WE, Carey RP 2002 Spinal Surgery and Severe Vitamin D Deficiency. MJA; May 6; 176:438–439

Plotnikoff GA, Quigley JM 2003 Prevalence of Severe Hypovitaminosis D in Patients with Persistent, Nonspecific Musculoskeletal Pain. Mayo Clin Proc 78:1463–1470

Prabhala A, Garg R, Dandona P 2000 Severe Myopathy Associated with Vitamin D Deficiency in Western New York. Arch Intern Med; April 24; 160:1199–1203

Schwalfenberg G 2009 Improvement of Chronic Back Pain of Failed Back Surgery with Vitamin D Repletion: A Case Series. J Am Board Fam Med 22:69–74

Turner MK, Hooten MH, Schmidt JE, Kerkvliet JL, Townsend CO, Bruce BK 2008 Prevalence and Clinical Correlates of Vitamin D Inadequacy among Patients with Chronic Pain. Pain Medicine 9(8):979–984

Chapter 17 (Obesity)

Cantor I 2008 Shedding Light on Vitamin D and Integrative Oncology. Integrative Cancer Therapies 7(2):81–89

Holick MF 2002 Vitamin D: The Unappreciated D-lightful Hormone that is Important for Skeletal and Cellular Health. Current Opinion in Endocrinology & Diabetes 9:87–98

Holick MF 2004 Vitamin D: Importance in the Prevention of Cancers, Type 1 Diabetes, Heart Disease, and Osteoporosis. American Journal of Clinical Nutrition; March; 79(3):362–371

Parikh SJ, Edelman M, Uwaifo GI, Freedman RJ, Semega-Janneh M, Reynolds J, Yanovski JA 2004 The Relationship between Obesity and Serum 1,25-Dihydroxy Vitamin D Concentrations in Healthy Adults. The Journal of Endocrinology & Metabolism 89(3):1196–1199

Chapter 18 (Spare the children)

American Diabetes Association 2010 Type 1 Diabetes Mortality Rates Dropping; November 10; www.diabetes.org

Dror DK, Allen LH 2010 Vitamin D Inadequacy in Pregnancy: Biology, Outcomes, and Interventions. Nutrition Reviews 68(8):465–477

Gale E 2002 The Rise of Childhood Type 1 Diabetes in the 20th Century. Diabetes 51:3353–3361

Grundmann M, von Versen-Höynck F 2011 Vitamin D—Roles in Woman's Reproductive Health? Reproductive Biology and Endocrinology 9:146

Holick MF 2004 Vitamin D: Importance in the Prevention of Cancers, Type 1 Diabetes, Heart Disease, and Osteoporosis. American Journal of Clinical Nutrition; March; 79(3):362–371

Holick MF 2006 Resurrection of Vitamin D Deficiency and Rickets. The Journal of Clinical Investigation 116(16):2062–2072

Hollis BW 2007 Vitamin D Requirements During Pregnancy and Lactation. Journal of Bone and Mineral Research 22(Suppl 2):V39–V44

Hollis BW, Wagner Cl 2004 Vitamin D Requirements during Lactation: High-Dose Maternal Supplementation as Therapy to Prevent Hypovitaminosis D for Both the Mother and the Nursing Infant. Am J Clin Nutr 80(Suppl):1752S–1758S

Hollis BW, Wagner CL 2006a Nutritional Vitamin D Status during Pregnancy: Reasons for Concern. CMAJ; April 25; 174(9):1287–1290

Hollis BW, Wagner CL 2006b Vitamin D Deficiency during Pregnancy: An Ongoing Epidemic. Am J Clin Nutr 84:273

Kjos SL, Buchanan TA 1999 Gestational Diabetes Mellitus. NEJM 341(23):1749–1756

Munns C, Zacharin MR, Rodda CP, Batch JA, Morley R, Cranswick NE, Craig ME, et al 2006 Prevention and Treatment of Infant and Childhood Vitamin D Deficiency in Australia and New Zealand: A Consensus Statement. MJA 185:268–272

Pappa HM, Gordon CM, Saslowsky TM, Zholudev A, Horr B, Shih M-C, Grand RJ 2006 Vitamin D Status in Children and Young Adults with Inflammatory Bowel Disease. Pediatrics; November; 118(5):1950–1961

Ponder SW, Sulivan S, McBath G 2000 Type 2 Diabetes Mellitus in Teens. Diabetes Spectrum 13(2):95

Sentonga TA, Semaeo EJ, Stettler N, Piccoli DA, Stallings VA, Zemel BS 2002 Vitamin D Status in Children, Adolescents, and Young Adults with Crohn's Disease. Am J Clin Nutr 76:1077–1081

Shin JS, Choi MY, Longtine MS, Nelson M 2020 Vitamin D Effects on Pregnancy and the Placenta. Placenta; December; 31(12):1027–1034

Wagner CL, Taylor SN, Hollis BW 2008 Does Vitamin D Make the World Go "Round"? Breastfeeding Medicine 3(4):239–250

Yorifuji J, Yorifuji T, Tachibana K, Nagai S, Kawai M, Momoi T, Nagasaka H, Hitayama H, Nakahata T 2008 Craniotabes in Normal Newborns: The Earliest Sign of Subclinical Vitamin D Deficiency. J Clin Endocrinol Metab 93:1784–1788

Chapter 19 (Now look here!)

Parekh N, Chappell RJ, Millen AE, Albert DM, Mares JA 2007 Association Between Vitamin D and Age-Related Macular Degeneration in the Third National Health and Nutrition Examination Survey, 1988 Through 1994. Arch Opthalmol; May; 125:661–669

Chapter 20 (Kidney Failure)

Al-Bar W, Martin KJ 2008 Vitamin D and Kidney Disease. Clin J Am Nephrol 3:1555–1560

Badalian SS, Rosenbaum PF 2010 Vitamin D and Pelvic Floor Disorders in Women. Obstetrics & Gynecology; April; 115(4):795–803

Boudville NC, Hodsman AB 2006 Renal Function and 25-hydroxyvitamin D Concentrations Predict Parathyroid Hormone Levels in Renal Transplant Patients. Nephrol Dial Transplant 21:2621–2624

Coli E, Rigatti P, Montorsi F, Artibani W, Petta S, Mondaini N, Scarpa R, et al 2006 BXL628, A Novel Vitamin D3 Analog Arrests Prostate Hyperplasia: A Randomized Clinical Trial. European Urology 49(2006):82–86

Ewers B, Gasbjerg A, Moelgaard C, Frederiksen AM, Marckmann P 2008 Vitamin D Status in Kidney Transplant Patients: Need for Intensified Routine Supplementation. Am J Clin Nutr 87:431–437

Kang H-T, Kim J-K, Shim J-Y, Lee H-R, Linton JA, Lee Y-J 2012 Low-Grade Inflammation, Metabolic Syndrome and the Risk of Chronic Kidney Disease: The 2005 Korean National Health and Nutrition Examination Survey. J Korean Med Sci 27:630–635

Li YC 2010 Renoprotective Effects of Vitamin D Analogs. Kidney International 78:134–139

Manchanda PK, Kibler AJ, Zhang M, Ravi J, Bid HK 2012 Vitamin D Receptor as a Therapeutic Target for Benign Prostatic Hyperplasia. Indian J Urol; Oct-Dec; 28(4):377–381

Parker-Autry CY, Burgio KL, Richter HE 2012 Vitamin D Status—A Clinical Review with Implications for the Pelvic Floor. Int Urogynecol J; November; 23(11):1517–1526

Querings K, Girndt M, Geisel J, Georg T, Tilgen W, Reichrath J 2006 25-Hydroxyvitamin D Deficiency in Renal Transplant Patients. J Clin Endocrinol Metab 91:526–529

Sorenson MB, Grant WB 2012 Does Vitamin D Deficiency Contribute to Erectile Dysfunction. Dermato-Endocrinology; April/May/June; 4(2):128–136

Tang J 2009 Vitamin D and Its Role in Chronic Kidney Disease 7(3)

Tang J, Yan H, Zhuang S 2012 Inflammation and Oxidative Stress in Obesity-Related Glomerulopathy. 2012:Article ID 608397

Williams S, Malatesta K, Norris K 2009 Vitamin D and Chronic Kidney Disease. Ethn Dis 19(4 Suppl 5):S5—8–11

Zehnder D, Quinkler M, Eardley KS, Bland R, Lepenies J, Hughes SV, Raymond NT, et al 2008 Reduction of the Vitamin D Hormonal System in Kidney Disease is Associated with Increased Renal Inflammation. Kidney International; November; 74(10):1334–1353

Chapter 21 (Areas of controversy and concern)

American Academy of Dermatology 2009 *Position Statement on Vitamin D.* http://www.aad.org/forms/policies/uploads/ps/ps-vitamin%20d.pdf

Bikle D 2009 Nonclassic Actions of Vitamin D. J Clin Endocrinol Metab 94:26–34

Grant WB 2011 The Institute of Medicine Did Not Find the Vtiamin D–Cancer Link Because it Ignored UV-B Dose Studies. Public Health Nutr; April; 14(4):745–746

Holick MF 2003 Vitamin D Deficiency: What a Pain It Is. Mayo Clin Proc 78:1457–1459

Holick MF 2005 The Vitamin D Epidemic and Its Health Consequences. J. Nutr. 135:2739S–2748S

Holick MF 2006a High Prevalence of Vitamin D Inadequacy and Implications for Health. Mayoclinicproceedings.com

Holick MF 2006b Resurrection of Vitamin D Deficiency and Rickets. The Journal of Clinical Investigation 116(16):2062–2072

Holick MF 2008 Vitamin D: A D-lightful Health Perspective. Nutrition Reviews 66(Suppl 2):S182–S194

Holick MF 2011 The D-batable Institute of Medicine Report: A D-lightful Perspective. Endocrine Practice; January/February; 17(1):143–149

Hollis BW, Wagner CI 2004 Vitamin D Requirements during Lactation: High-Dose Maternal Supplementation as Therapy to Prevent Hypovitaminosis D for Both the Mother and the Nursing Infant. Am J Clin Nutr 80(Suppl):1752S–1758S

Reichrath J 2007 Vitamin D and the Skin: An Ancient Friend, Revisited. Experimental Dermatology 16:618–625

Chapter 22 (Be safe out there)

Armas LA, Hollis BW, Heaney RP 2004 Vitamin D_2 is Much Less Effective than Vitamin D_3 in Humans. J Clin Endocrinol Metab 89:5387–5391

Heaney RF 2008 Vitamin D in Health and Disease. Clin J Am Soc Nephrol 3:1535–1541

Holick MF 2010 The Vitamin D Deficiency Pandemic: A Forgotten Hormone Important for Health. Public Health Reviews 32(1):267–283

Holick MF 2011 The D-batable Institute of Medicine Report: A D-lightful Perspective. Endocrine Practice; January/February; 17(1):143–149

Hollis BW, Wagner Cl 2004 Vitamin D Requirements during Lactation: High-Dose Maternal Supplementation as Therapy to prevent Hypovitaminosis D for Both the Mother and the Nursing Infant. Am J Clin Nutr 80(Suppl):1752S–1758S

Krasowski MD 2011 Pathology Consultation on Vitamin D Testing. Am J Clin Pathol 136:507–514

Misra M, Pacaud D, Petryk A, Collett-Solberg PF, Kappy M 2008 Vitamin D Deficiency in Children and its Management: Review of Current Knowledge and Recommendations. Pediatrics 122:398–417

Chapter 23 (Recommendations)

Arnson Y, Amital H, Shoenfeld Y 2007 Vitamin D and Autoimmunity: New Aetiological and Therapeutic Considerations. Ann Rheum Dis; June 8; 0:1–6

Brot C, Jorgensen NR, Sorensen OH 1999 The Influence of Smoking in Vitamin D Status and Calcium. European Journal of Clinical Nutrition 53:920–925

Cantorna MT 2000 Vitamin D and Autoimmunity: Is Vitamin D Status an Environmental Factor Affecting Autoimmune Disease Prevalence? Proceedings of the Society for Experimental Biology and Medicine 223:230–233

Dawodu A, Wagner CL 2007 Mother-Child Vitamin D Deficiency: An International Perspective. Arch Dis Child 92:737–740

DeLuca H 2004 Overview of General Physiological Features and Functions of Vitamin D. Am J Clin Nutr 80(Suppl):1689S–1696S

Fakih MG, Trump DL, Johnson CS, Tian L, Muindi J, Sunga AY 2009 Chemotherapy is Linked to Severe Vitamin D Deficiency in Patients with Colorectal Cancer. Int J Colorectal Dis 24:219–224

Giovannucci E 2009 Expanding Roles of Vitamin D. J Clin Endocrinol Metab; February; 94(2):418–420

Holick MF 2002 Vitamin D: The Unappreciated D-lightful Hormone that is Important for Skeletal and Cellular Health. Current Opinion in Endocrinology & Diabetes 9:87–98

Holick MF 2003a Vitamin D: A Millenium Perspective. Journal of Cellular Biochemistry 88:296–307

Holick MF 2003b Vitamin D Deficiency: What a Pain It Is. Mayo Clin Proc 78:1457–1459

Holick MF 2004a Vitamin D: Importance in the Prevention of Cancers, Type 1 Diabetes, Heart Disease, and Osteoporosis. American Journal of Clinical Nutrition; March; 79(3):362–371

Holick MF 2004b Sunlight and Vitamin D for Bone Health and Prevention of Autoimmune Diseases, Cancers, and Cardiovascular Disease. American Journal of Clinical Nutrition; December; 80(6):1678S–1688S

Holick MF 2005 The Vitamin D Epidemic and Its Health Consequences. J. Nutr. 135:2739S–2748S

Holick MF 2006 High Prevalence of Vitamin D Inadequacy and Implications for Health. Mayoclinicproceedings.com

Holick MF 2011 The D-batable Institute of Medicine Report: A D-lightful Perspective. Endocrine Practice; January/February; 17(1):143–149

Hollis BW 2007 Vitamin D Requirements During Pregnancy and Lactation. Journal of Bone and Mineral Research 22(Suppl 2):V39–V44

Hollis BW, Wagner CI 2006 Vitamin D Requirements during Lactation: High-Dose Maternal Supplementation as Therapy to Prevent Hypovitaminosis D for Both the Mother and the Nursing Infant. Am J Clin Nutr 80(Suppl):1752S–1758S

Huisman AM, White KP, Algra A, Harth M, Vieth R, Jacobs J, Bulsma J, Bell DA 2001 Vitamin D Levels in Women with Systemic Lupus Erthematosus and Fibromyalgia. J Rheumatol 28:2535–2539

Kahn QJ, Fabian CJ 2010 How I Treat Vitamin D Deficiency. Journal of Oncology Practice 6(2):97–101

Koutkia P, Lu Z, Chen TC, Holick MF 2001 Treatment of Vitamin D Deficiency Due to Crohn's Disease with Tanning Bed Ultraviolet B Radiation. Gastroenterology 122:1485–1488

Lee JH, O'Keefe JH, Bell D, Hensrud DD, Holick MF 2008 Vitamin D Deficiency: An Important, Common, and Early Treatable Cardiovascular Risk Factor. Journal of the American College of Cardiology 52(24):1949–1956

Leventis P, Patel S 2008 Clinical Aspects of Vitamin D in the Management of Rheumatoid Arthritis. Rheumatology 47:1617–1621

Mann D 2005 Vitamin D Status More Important than High Calcium Intake for Calcium Homeostasis. Endotext.org

Mulligan BG, Licata A 2010 Taking Vitamin D With the Largest Meal Improves Absorption and Results in Higher Serum Levels of 25-Hydroxyvitamin D. Journal of Bone and Mineral Research; April; 25(4):928–930

Norman AW 2008 From Vitamin D to Hormone D: Fundamentals of the Vitamin D Endocrine System Essential for Good Health. Am J Clin Nutr 88(Suppl):491S–499S

Schwalfenberg G 2007 Not Enough Vitamin D: Health Consequences for Canadians. Canadian Family Medicine 53:842–854

Tangpricha V, Turner A, Spina C, Decastro S, Chen TC, Holick MF 2004 Tanning is Associated with Optimal Vitamin D Status (Serum 25-hydroyvitamin D Concentration) and Higher Bone Mineral Density. Am J Clin Nutr 80:1645–1649

Tuohy K, Steinman TI 2005 Hypercalcemia Due to Excess 1,25-Dihydroxyvitamin D in Crohn's Disease. American Journal of Kidney Diseases 45(1):e3–e6

Vieth R 1999 Vitamin D Supplementation, 25-hydroxyvitamin D Concentrations, and Safety. American Journal of Clinical Nutrition 69(5):842–856

Wagner CL, Taylor SN, Hollis BW 2008 Does Vitamin D Make the World Go "Round"? Breastfeeding Medicine 3(4):239–250

WebMD 2008 Arthritis: Disease-Modifying Medications; July 30

Zittermann A, Schleithoff SS, Tenderich G, Berthold HK, Körfer R, Stehle P 2003 Low Vitamin D Status: A Contributing Factor in the Pathogenesis of Congestive Heart Failure? J Am Coll Cardiol 41:105–112

Conclusion

Al Faraj SA, Al Mutairi JA 2003 Vitamin D Deficiency and Chronic Low Back Pain in Saudi Arabia. Spine 28:177–179

Cui Y, Rohan TE 2006 Vitamin D, Calcium, and Breast Cancer Risk: A Review. Cancer Epidemiol Biomarkers Prev 15(18):1427–1437

Holick MF 2003 Vitamin D: A Millenium Perspective. Journal of Cellular Biochemistry 88:296–307

Holick MF 2008 Vitamin D: A D-lightful Health Perspective. Nutrition Reviews 66(Suppl 2):S182–S194

Spina CS, Tangpricha V, Uskokovic M, Adorinic L, Maehr H, Holick MF 2006 Vitamin D and Cancer. Anticancer Research 26:2515–2524

Welsh J 2007 Vitamin D and Prevention of Breast Cancer. Acta Pharmacol Sin; September; 28(9):1373–1382

www.ingramcontent.com/pod-product-compliance
Lightning Source LLC
Chambersburg PA
CBHW030841210326
41521CB00025B/520